Dynamic Aspects of
BRAIN SCANNING

JYOJI HANDA, M.D.

Instructor, Department of Neurosurgery, Kyoto University Medical School
Kyoto, Japan

UNIVERSITY PARK PRESS

Baltimore and London

Library of Congress Cataloging in Publication Data

Handa, Jyoji.
    Dynamic aspects of brain scanning.

    Bibliography: p.
    1. Brain—Diseases—Diagnosis. I. Title.
II. Title: Brain scanning. DNLM: 1. Brain diseases
—Radiography. 2. Radioisotope scanning. WL 141 H236d
  1972
RC386.5.H36   616.8′04′75   72-7259
ISBN 0-8391-0733-1

PUBLISHERS
© American Edition, 1972 by IGAKU SHOIN LTD., 5-29-11 Hongo Bunkyo-ku, Tokyo.
    Rights in the United States of America and the Dominion of Canada granted to
    UNIVERSITY PARK PRESS: Chamber of Commerce Building
                      Baltimore, Maryland 21202

Printed and Bound in Japan

FOREWORD

Classical neuroradiology, which in the past has been primarily morphologically oriented, has in the last years included more and more dynamic angiographic studies with a consequent enhancement of its diagnostic possibilities. The diagnosis of cerebro-vascular diseases has particularly benefited by this current trend. Functional tests, that is those dynamic studies done with altered blood gasses or change in the blood pressure, reveal even more about the autoregulatory mechanisms.

Thanks to the discovery of new isotopes and the improvement in instrumentation, scanning techniques and data processing, scintigraphy has likewise made the meaningful step from a pure morphologic diagnosis, that is the localization of a circumscribed lesion based on the differential isotope uptake between normal and pathologic tissues, to the dynamic radioangiography which demonstrates circulatory disturbances and the activity-time relationships in pathologic processes. In many cases this enables a more precise diagnosis than that previously possible. Thus, the scintigraphy has been elevated to a level comparable with the X-ray examination. The critical evaluation of the results of both examinations enables the diagnostician to confirm, improve or disprove a doubtful diagnosis.

With his outstanding knowledge of brain circulation and classical neuroradiological techniques, Dr. J. Handa has been able to apply the functional aspects of the radio-logic examination to the scintigraphic method. As an experienced neurosurgeon he is well able to separate the practical, important and confirmed from the hypothetical. He is not interested in playing one method against the other but attempts to define a practical, useful combination of the two. In his well written, understandable mono-graph, he has critically reviewed the voluminous literature and combined this laborious study with his own great experience in the interpretation of dynamic brain scintigraphy.

His monograph is of greatest interest to the clinician who must be familiar enough with both methods to use them in his daily work. This monograph is certain to receive its well deserved acknowledgement. I hope it will be able to overcome the lasting resistance against the combined interpretation of brain diseases using both neuroradiologic and scintigraphic techniques.

November 1971

P. Huber

Berne/Switzerland

ACKNOWLEDGEMENTS

I would like to thank Dr. C. Araki, Emeritus Professor, and Dr. H. Handa, Professor, of the Department of Neurosurgery, Kyoto University Medical School, for their supports and encouragements throughout the present study.

I am greatly indebted to Dr. Peter Huber, Professor of Neuroradiology, Inselspital, Berne, Switzerland, for having introduced me to the field of diagnostic neuroradiology, and to Dr. John S. Meyer, Professor of Neurology, Baylor College of Medicine, Houston, Texas, for having provided me with the opportunity of studying in his laboratory. Dr. Huber has kindly sent me his own materials for illustrating Chapter V (Figures 16 through 19).

I am very grateful to Dr. K. Torizuka and Dr. K. Hamamoto, of the Central Clinical Radioisotope Division for their generous help and cooperation. I must particularly acknowledge the contribution of Miss T. Kousaka, Chief Technician of the Radioisotope Division and the Nursing Staff of the Department of Neurosurgery; without their patient and skillful cooperation, many of the long and tedious studies could never have been completed.

Last but not least, the author would like to thank sincerely the publisher, Igaku Shoin Ltd., for their full cooperation at all times.

J. H.

CONTENTS

INTRODUCTION

Since Moore's original report [105] in 1948 that the brain tumors accumulate radio-active substances which are excluded from the normal brain tissue, many hundreds of reports have appeared in the world literature on the radioisotopic localization of intracranial lesions. Particularly during the past decade, enormous advances have been made in refinement of instrumentation, in improvement of scanning technic and data processing, and in development of appropriate radionuclide preparations with a short half-life, and at present brain scanning has become the reliable diagnostic tool which is indispensable for the daily practice in neurologic-neurosurgical service.

Even with present day instrumentation and radionuclide, the diagnostic accuracy of brain scanning still does not reach that of angiography or air study, and brain scanning at the present time apparently does not replace other neuroradiologic examinations. However, brain scanning is quite safe and not uncomfortable to the patient, it spares the patient morbidity and mortality which, though rare, are inevitable with the use of most of the radiologic contrast studies of the brain. Brain scanning can be performed easily on an out-patient basis, it is safe even in infants or acutely ill patients. It can be used for screening purposes in the patients suspected of harboring intracranial diseases, and it can be repeated at varying intervals after operation or irradiation therapy for the purpose of early detection of recurrent tumors with the negligible radiation exposure. Three dimensional isotopic images make the target setting more accurate for irradiation of intracranial tumors.

In this volume, our experience of brain scanning performed over the past four years is summarized, and its dynamic aspects are stressed. Most of the studies were performed with a gamma-ray scintillation camera (Pho/Gamma III, Nuclear Chicago). The use of a gamma-ray scintillation camera and a short-lived radionuclide such as ^{99m}Tc pertechnetate permits the dynamic study of an isotope bolus as it traverses the normal and pathologic focus in the brain. Vascular phases of the scintigrams are stored and replayed by the use of a video-tape system. Following this vascular phase, time-lapse scintiphotography and the use of a memory system make possible the visual and digital assessments of the time course of isotope uptake in multiple areas in the brain. In addition to the morphological images of brain scan such as the location, size, shape, density, margin, homogeneity and multiplicity of the radioactive foci, such a dynamic approach has substantially improved the diagnostic accuracy and has provided further useful informations as to the nature of the lesion [52, 57].

More recently we have employed a gamma-ray scintillation camera for the purpose of blood flow and perfusion analysis of the brain. Although they are still in the experimental stage, these studies have often proved to be a useful adjunctive technic in the examination of selected patients with difficult diagnostic problems.

Chapter I

BASIC MECHANISM AND TECHNICAL ASPECT OF BRAIN SCANNING

1. *Basic Mechanism of Positive Scan*

Positive result in brain scanning depends upon a focal accumulation of radionuclide at the site of the pathology, and a resultant achievement of a certain level of lesion-to-brain concentration gradient of radionuclide.

No substance has ever been found to achieve a focal concentration exceeding that of the initial blood level, and the seemingly selective focal accumulation is due to the low background activity in the normal brain [5].

It has been frequently suggested that the mechanism of the positive scan, or of the high lesion-to-brain uptake ratio, is the focal absence or the impaired function of the blood-brain-barrier. The blood-brain-barrier is generally considered to be a hypothetical structure or functional mechanism consisting of multitudes of membranes and a number of enzyme actions. Although there are many examples of alteration in permeability of the blood-brain-barrier in neoplastic, vascular, traumatic, inflammatory or degenerative diseases of the brain, only few of them have been studied adequately, and many other factors must be considered to be responsible for the selective uptake of the radionuclides, including the blood contents of the pathologic lesion [121], abnormal structure of the neoplastic blood vessels [38, 108, 120], respective size of the extracellular spaces [38, 67], pinocytosis [76], carrier transport [80], passive diffusion through the membrane system of the brain, and several others. Contribution of each of these factors seems to differ among the various types of lesions and from one tracer agent to the other. As far as the short-lived radionuclide such as ^{99m}Tc pertechnetate is used for scanning purposes, the factor of blood content in the lesion seems to play a very important role, as the scanning is performed shortly after administration of the tracer while the blood level is still very high [52].

Metabolic factors might also be responsible for the accumulation in the tumor of several kinds of radioactive substances, such as seen with ^{131}I RISA in cerebral metastases of thyroid cancer or with labeled chloroquine analogue in melanomas [7, 9]. The study has been continued by several investigators to compare the selective uptake of the radionuclides with different chemical properties by various lesions, in an attempt to find the criteria for selecting the adequate tracer agent with high specific affinity to a given lesion [31, 88, 146, 147]. Although the results are so far largely non-productive, DiChiro and coworkers [31] have suggested the possibility of a "relative" specificity for certain tracers to some types of the pathologies (^{131}I RISA for cerebral metastases, [197]Hg and [203]Hg chlormerodrin for glioma group, ^{131}I AF for sarcoma). Immunologic approach seems to be an another promising possibility for finding tracer with a specific affinity for various kinds of tumors [8].

2. Radioactive Agents for Brain Scanning

The ideal radionuclide for brain scanning should satisfy the following prerequisites;

1) The isotope should be rapidly cleared of the blood, and its biological half-life should be short. The agent without specific affinity to any special organ is desirable.

2) The isotope should be picked up preferentially by the tumor or other pathologic tissue with a minimum degree of uptake in the surrounding normal brain tissue, since the high lesion-to-brain uptake ratio is the important factor for successful scan.

3) The isotope should have a physical half-life short enough to reduce the whole body irradiation to the minimum. On the other hand, if the half-life is too short, the shelf life makes the stock impossible. At the present time, a physical half-life of two to three days seems to be desirable for a laboratory of small size, but a half-life of several hours from the feeder system (cow) may be more ideal.

4) The isotope should be a pure monoenergetic gamma-ray emitter, since the beta radiation enhances the irradiation but does not contribute to the external detection of the lesion. The energy level of the gamma radiation between 80–250 KeV is ideal for the collimation and external detection by the present day instrumentation.

5) Preparation should be easily synthesized with a high specific activity. It should be chemically nontoxic and pyrogen-free.

Table 1 lists the preparations which are commonly used for the brain scanning, but none of them is really ideal. At the present time, most institutions use ^{99m}Tc pertechnetate and [197]Hg or [203]Hg chlormerodrin. We have used ^{99m}Tc pertechnetate almost exclusively for the brain scanning, because it can be administered in a large dose. The over-all resolution is better and the scanning time is shortened, so that the sequential study is easily performed. More recently, [169]Yb DTPA has become commercially available, which seems to be useful because of a short biological half-life and pretty long physical half-life (Table 1). Scan images with [169]Yb DTPA are much the same as those with ^{99m}Tc pertechnetate [40, 66, 153, 154].

3. Scanning Instruments

Brain scanning is essentially a technic for displaying the distribution of radioactivity throughout the head. In the original work of Moore [105], a Geiger-Müller counter was used for this purpose. The count rates were determined at multiple sites over the head and their distribution was compared. A few years later, a scintillation counter was introduced for this counting purpose. The procedure was fairly accurate in the hands of well-trained personnel, but it was time-consuming and impractical for examinations of a large number of patients.

Until recently most laboratories used the mechanical scanner of one type or another. They were equipped with NaI (Tl-activated) crystal and the data were displayed on a sheet of paper, photographic film or the imaging screen.

Recently, stationary detector system has been developed. They consist of a large single NaI crystal of 10–13 inches in diameter, or a battery of multiple small crystals, or a x-ray intensifier system. By use of these new devices, imaging of the

Table 1 Representative radionuclides used routinely for brain scanning

Radio-nuclide	Compound	Usual dose and route	Physical half-life	Beta emmi-sion	Gamma energy	Blood clearance half-life	Target organ and dose per scan	
^{169}Yb	DTPA	10 mCi i.v.	32 days	Yes	63, 110, 131, 177, 198, 308 KeV	10 hr.	Bladder	3 rads
^{99m}Tc	Pertech-netate	10 mCi i.v., oral	6 hr.	No	140 KeV	5.5 hr.	Bowel	1 rad
^{113m}In	FeDTPA	10 mCi i.v.	1.7 hr.	No	390 KeV	40 min.	Blood	500 mr
^{197}Hg	Chlormer-odrin	10 μCi/kg i.v.	65 hr.	No	77 KeV	4 hr.	Kidney	24 rads
^{203}Hg	Chlormer-odrin	10 μCi/kg i.v.	46 days	Yes	279 KeV	4 hr.	Kidney	38–115 rads
^{131}I	Serum Albumin	5 μCi/kg i.v.	8 days	Yes	364 KeV	ca 48 hr.	Blood	2.5 rads
^{131}I	Polyvinyl Pyrrolidone	500 μCi i.v.	8 days	Yes	364 KeV	ca 8 hr.	Total Body Liver	550 mr 25 rads
^{74}As	Arsenate	1.3 mCi i.v.	17.5 days	Yes	Positron. 511 KeV	very rapid	Kidney	7.2 rads
^{64}Cu	DTPA	2 mCi i.v.	12.8 hr.	Yes	Positron. 511 KeV	ca 10 min.	Liver	3.2 rads
^{68}Ga	EDTA	400–500 μCi i.v	68 min.	No	Positron. 511 KeV	ca 2 hr.	Kidney	150 mr

radioisotopic distribution in the organ is obtained very rapidly and the sequential study can be performed accurately. Our study has been done almost exclusively with the Anger type gamma-ray scintillation camera, with the exception of ^{131}I MAA perfusion scanning and several others.

Chapter II

POSITIONING OF HEAD, NORMAL SCINTIGRAPHIC ANATOMY, NORMAL VARIANTS AND ARTEFACT

1. *Frontal or Anterior View*

In this text, the scintigram taken with the detector positioned over the face or the forehead is called the "*frontal*" or "*anterior*" view to avoid confusion. It is sometimes named "*antero-posterior*" view or "*a.-p.*" view, however, the antero-posterior view in common radiologic terminology means a picture taken with the anterior-posteriorly travelling beam and the film facing the occiput.

Similarly, the scintigram taken with the probe positioned over the occiput is called the "*occipital*" or "*posterior*" view.

For the frontal view, the patient is placed supine and the detector head is placed over the face so that the canthomeatal line is perpendicular to the detector surface (Figure 1).

When ^{99m}Tc pertechnetate is used as a tracer, the tissue with high vascularity and blood content shows an increased radioactivity. In the frontal view, the normal brain

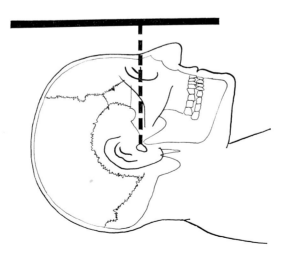

Fig. 1 Positioning in frontal view.

tissue appears as areas of low background activity separated into two halves by a midline ridge of increased activity. This midline activity tends to become widened superiorly and represents midline vascular structures, such as the anterior portion of the superior sagittal sinus and the anterior cerebral artery. At the vertex the superior sagittal sinus is seen end-on, in the configuration of an inverted triangle.

A uniform peripheral band represents the scalp, skull bone and the blood vessels of the meninges. Lower portion of the peripheral rim widens medially, representing the radioactivity in the temporalis muscle and the sylvian vessels.

Along the skull base, there is noted an area of high radioactivity in the midline due to nasal mucosa and sphenoid and ethmoid sinuses. Orbits are seen as areas of less density on both sides. More inferiorly the parotid gland, maxillary sinus and oropharynx appear as dense areas of high radioactivity (Figure 2).

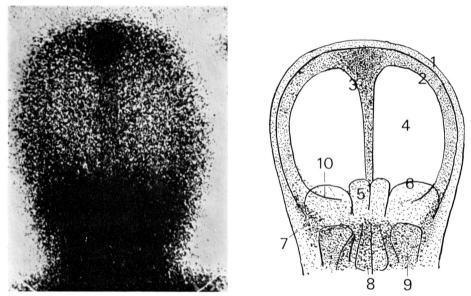

Fig. 2 Normal frontal scintigram. *1.* Scalp activity; *2.* Skull and cortical vessels; *3.* Superior sagittal sinus; *4.* Cerebral hemisphere; *5.* Frontal sinus; *6.* Orbital area; *7.* Parotid gland activity; *8.* Nasal mucosa; *9.* Maxillary sinus; and *10.* Floor of anterior cranial fossa.

When the head is rotated to the one side in the frontal or occipital view, the peripheral rim activity becomes asymmetrical and may simulate a pathologic condition, such as the chronic subdural hematoma. The midline zone of increased activity in this case loses its lineality and midline location.

2. *"en face"* View

For the *"en face"* view of Wilson and Briggs [163], the canthomeatal line is angulated by 15–20 degrees to the cephalad direction and the detector surface is placed parallel to the horizontal table top (Figure 3).

In this view, an area of high radioactivity is seen in the midline, representing the mucous membrane of nose, pharynx and oral cavity. Parotid glands are projected

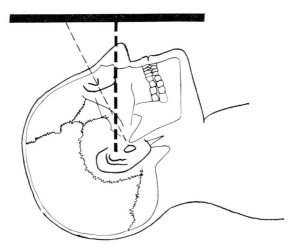

Fig. 3 Positioning in "en face" view.

more inferiorly. Radiating outward and upward from the midline activity toward the temporalis muscle activity is an another linear radioactive zone, which is due to the sphenoparietal sinus and the sylvian vessels. Between this linear activity and the parotid gland activity lies the rather cool area representing the orbit and through this orbital area, lesion in the anterior portion of the middle fossa or the orbital pathology is detected (Figure 4).

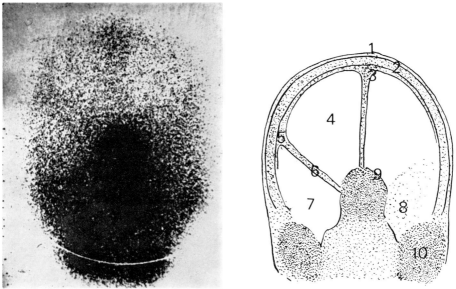

Fig. 4 Scintigram in en face view. *1.* Scalp activity; *2.* Skull; *3.* Superior sagittal sinus; *4.* Cerebral hemisphere; *5.* Temporalis muscle; *6.* Sphenoid wing and middle cerebral artery; *7.* Orbital area and anterior temporal region. *8.* Abnormal uptake of retro-orbital sarcoma; *9.* Nasopharynx and paranasal air sinuses; and *10.* Parotid gland.

The use of "*en face*" view is helpful in studying the anterior temporal lesion. This area is frequently obscured in the conventional frontal view, and is difficult to visualize in the lateral view because of high radioactivity of the overlying temporalis muscle. Also lesions in the orbit, and the pathologic process of the sphenoid bone are well shown in this view. Detection of the lesions in the suprasellar or olfactory region, on the contrary, tends to be difficult in this view.

3. *Posterior or Occipital View*

The normal brain tissue appears as the symmetrical areas of low background activity separated in the midline by the radioactivity of posterior portion of the superior sagittal sinus in the occipital or posterior view (Figure 5).

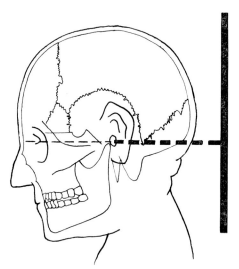

Fig. 5   Positioning in occipital view.

The peripheral activity is similar to that in the frontal view. The torcular Herophili is often seen as a localized, dense area of activity lying in the midline, from which arises the radioactivity of the transverse sinuses. The transverse sinuses are not necessarily symmetrical, and one side may be larger than the other, usually the right side being more prominent. Beneath the transverse sinuses the cerebellum is represented as an area of relatively low activity, which is often separated into halves by a thin band of increased activity due to the occipital sinus. Below the level of the transverse sinus, a peripheral rim widens medially, this being due to the sigmoid sinus activity (Figure 6).

In the interpretation of the occipital view, it is always important to check whether or not the posterior fossa is well visualized beneath the transverse sinuses. If the posterior fossa is not seen well, the occipital view should be repeated with the head well flexed (*Angled Posterior View*).

In the occipital view, motion of the head during scanning procedure or the faulty positioning of the head may result in an asymmetry in the background radioactivity of the cerebellar fossae, leading to an erroneous diagnosis of the posterior fossa mass lesion.

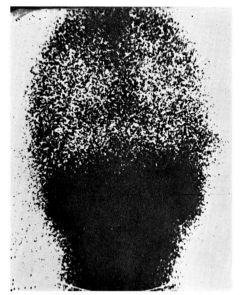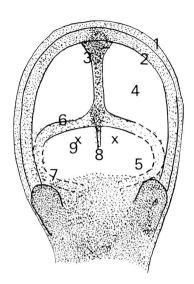

Fig. 6 Normal scintigram in occipital view. *1.* Scalp; *2.* Skull and cortical vessels; *3.* Superior sagittal sinus; *4.* Cerebral hemisphere; *5.* Cerebellar hemisphere; *6.* Transverse sinus; *7.* Sigmoid sinus; *8.* Occipital sinus; and *9.* Position of internal acoustic meatus.

4. Lateral View

For the lateral view, the head is rotated to right or left and the detector surface is positioned parallel to the midsagittal plane (Figure 7).

In the lateral view, radioactivities of the scalp, superior sagittal sinus and the large vessels of the meninges form a peripheral band around the cerebral hemispheres. This peripheral rim activity is thin anteriorly and becomes gradually thicker as it courses posteriorly toward the torcular Herophili, but in many cases the radioactivity once decreases in the region immediately above the torcular (Figure 8).

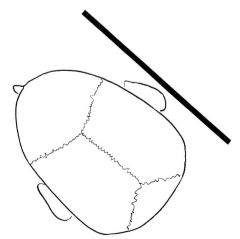

Fig. 7 Positioning in right lateral view.

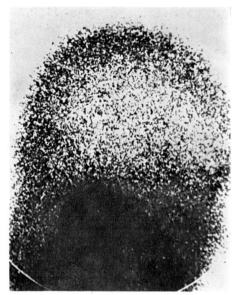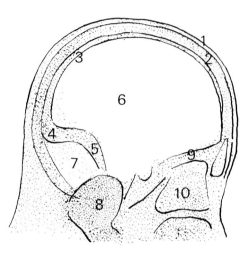

Fig. 8 Normal scintigram in right lateral view. *1.* Scalp; *2.* Skull; *3.* Superior sagittal sinus; *4.* Torcular Herophili; *5.* Sigmoid sinus; *6.* Cerebral hemisphere; *7.* Cerebellar hemisphere; *8.* Parotid gland; *9.* Floor of anterior cranial fossa; and *10.* Orbital area and paranasal sinuses.

When the skull is thick, peripheral rim may be seen in two layers, the outer one due to the scalp radioactivity and the inner one representing the radioactivity in the superior sagittal sinus and the large meningeal vessels. Occasionally, the peripheral rim normally thickens at the vertex in the rolandic region. When compared with the radiographs of the skull or the angiograms, this seems to be due to the large superficial cerebral veins and lacunar veins, and should be differentiated from the parasagittal mass.

The orbit is seen as an area of relatively low radioactivity which is demarcated from the frontal lobe by the floor of the anterior cranial fossa, the line of demarcation being perpendicular to the forehead. The activity of the skull base angles downward about 30 degrees at the junction of anterior and middle cranial fossae, and extends posteriorly to the base of the posterior fossa.

The posterior fossa is seen as an area of low radioactivity, limited postero-inferiorly by the activities of the occipital bone and nuchal muscles, antero-inferiorly by the skull base activities and superiorly by the superiorly convex radioactivities due to the transverse and sigmoid sinuses (Figure 11). The right and left lateral views should be the mirror images except for the activity of the transverse and sigmois sinuses.

The increased radioactivity beneath the orbit represents the nasal cavity, pharynx and oral cavity and the maxillary sinus. More posteriorly the activity of the mastoid cells and the parotid gland is seen.

Occasionally, a triangular area of increased radioactivity is seen emerging from the base of the skull at the junction of the anterior and middle cranial fossae. This is seen particularly when the scanning is performed immediately after administration of ^{99m}Tc pertechnetate and is due to radioactivity in the large arteries and veins in the sylvian region. This may simulate the suprasellar pathology such as the pituitary adenoma or meningioma of tuberculum sellae; however, those tumors are usually round or oval and persist longer in the sequential studies.

When the head is tilted toward or away from the detector surface, the lateral view is distorted and may be misleading. Particularly if the head is tilted toward the collimator surface, an unusual prominence of the activity of the base occurs in the sellar region, more or less simulating the picture of mass in the suprasellar region.

5. *Vertex View*

For the vertex view, the patient is placed prone with his head hyperextended so that the canthomeatal line is horizontal. The detector surface is positioned parallel to the canthomeatal line and the neck and back are shielded [64, 65]. (Figure 9).

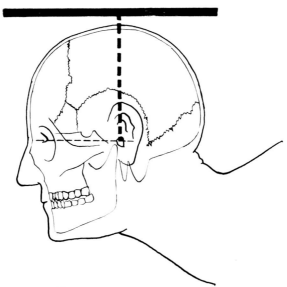

Fig. 9 Positioning in vertex view.

The oval outline of the head in the vertex view is formed by a peripheral rim which is thin anteriorly and becomes progressively thicker posteriorly, due to the radio-activity in the salivary glands and nuchal muscles. In the posterior portion the peripheral rim is occasionally thicker on the right side, probably due to the larger size of the transverse sinus on this side. The superior sagittal sinus is seen as a midline band of radioactivity; this also becomes broader as it courses posteriorly until it finally reaches the torcular Herophili, which is seen as a triangular area of increased radioactivity (Figure 10).

Occasionally a triangular area of isotope collection is seen in the anterior portion which represents the radioactivity in the nasal and oral cavities. One mg of atropine sulfate given intramuscularly reduces the oral and nasal secretion and minimizes the interference with scan interpretation [65].

6. *Choroid Plexus Activity*

When ^{99m}Tc pertechnetate scanning is carried out without premedication of the

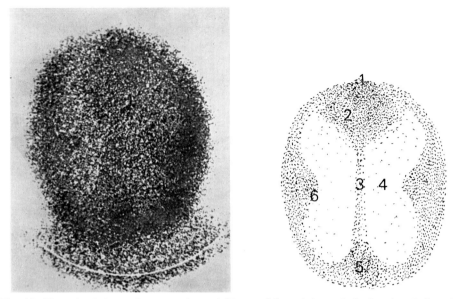

Fig. 10 Normal scintigram in vertex view. *1.* Nose and frontal sinus; *2.* Oral cavity; *3.* Superior sagittal sinus; *4.* Cerebral hemisphere; *5.* Torcular Herophili; and *6.* Temporalis muscle and parotid gland.

patients with atropine or potassium perchlorate, technetium concentrates in the choroid plexus of the lateral ventricles and the activity can be seen in the lateral view in about a half of cases [89, 164]. In five to 10 per cent of cases the activity is markedly high and causes confusion in scan interpretation (Figure 11). The accumulation of radioactivity in the choroid plexus can be abolished by an oral ad-

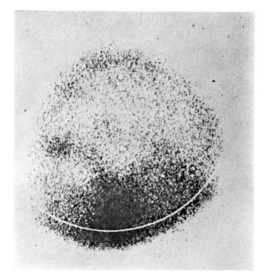

Fig. 11 Normal scintigram in right lateral view. Choroid plexus activity and dominant transverse sinus.

ministration of potassium perchlorate in a dosis of 200–400 mg in the adult of an average body weight 30 minutes prior to injection of the tracer. In doubtful cases, scanning should be repeated after blocking the plexus.

7. Artefact

Since ^{99m}Tc pertechnetate is secreted in the saliva and in the gastric juice, contamination from saliva or vomitus of the patient's hair, scalp or face occasionally shows a high radioactivity, and this may lead to serious misinterpretation of scan images. This should be particularly borne in mind since a number of cases sent for brain scanning have disturbance of consciousness and frequent vomiting.

Contamination of the examiner's finger may prove to be a rare source of error.

In infant, especially when hydrocephalic, injection of ^{99m}Tc pertechnetate into the scalp vein shows a clear radioactive focus in and around the site of injection. The extracranial location of activity can be easily seen in the multiple views, however, the tracer should not be given by this route in order to avoid misinterpretation. Even when the isotope is not given into the scalp vein, the radioactivity may accumulate locally in the scalp if the scalp vein has been used for the purpose of intravenous infusion of fluids or drugs.

Preceding carotid angiography or pneumoencephalography, in our experience, does not seem to significantly affect the scan results, although the radionuclide angiography performed immediately after injection of the contrast medium may occasionally show differences in hemispherical perfusion images.

Trephination of the skull for ventriculography or cerebrospinal fluid drainage, on the other hand, causes a misleading focal accumulation of radioactivity and it persists for several months after operation.

When the tracer is injected into the carotid artery for the purpose of radionuclide angiography, the cerebral hemisphere on the perfused side shows higher radioactivity and the asymmetry persists at least for one hour. Unilateral and diffuse increase in radioactivity may simulate the scan image of chronic subdural hematoma.

8. Calvarial and Scalp Lesions as a Source of Error

Abnormal radioisotope accumulation in the brain scan may be located in the brain, calvaria or the scalp. The localization of the area of abnormal radioisotope uptake is usually possible by examination of multiple views, but occasionally an abnormal uptake in the skull or the scalp may be difficult to differentiate from that inside the brain, and this may cause serious confusion in the interpretation of the brain scan. When an area of abnormal superficial uptake is noted in the brain scan, the scalp should be checked carefully for the presence of any signs of trauma or infection, and at the same time comparison with the adequate projection of the plain radiographs of the skull is indispensable.

Bruises, contusions and lacerations of the scalp and subgaleal hematoma accumulate radionuclide probably because of an increase in permeability of the damaged blood vessels. The surgical wound of the scalp also causes similar changes in the brain scan. The scintigram demonstrates a focal increase in the radioactivity of the peripheral rim. Those radioisotope accumulations subside spontaneously in several weeks to a few weeks, but as far as ^{99m}Tc pertechnetate is used, it seems that the radionuclide accumulation persists until long after the resolution of edema and other inflammatory changes of the wound.

Vascular lesion of the scalp such as angioma, or the infectious process of the scalp also accumulates the radionuclide, and recent irradiation with ^{60}Co or other high kilovoltage beams may show an area of increased radioactivity.

Following the craniotomy, an area of abnormal radionuclide accumulation at the site of operation persists for several months. Although its superficial position is usually detected easily by comparing the multiple views, it may become a source of confusion in the follow-up scanning for possible recurrences in brain tumor cases. In the post-craniotomy scan, superficial abnormal radionuclide accumulation may be in part due to the reactive formation of the bone, however, the most of the radionuclide accumulation is due to an increased permeability and proliferation of the scalp and dural vessels, and granulation tissue of meningeal origin. Replacement or permanent removal of the reflected bone flap does not cause any significant difference in the postoperative scintigrams, except for a possible change in configuration of the calvaria after removal of the flap.

Chapter III

TRAUMATIC CONDITIONS

1. Chronic Subdural Hematoma

The chronic subdural hematomas, either of traumatic origin or without the history of preceding head injury, are detected with high accuracy by brain scanning. Our experience in more than 20 adult cases shows 100 per cent detection accuracy, and we consider the scanning as an important study in patients complaining of prolonged or recurred headache or other nonspecific symptoms after trivial head injury.

The lesion is characteristically shown as an asymmetrical, crescent-shaped radioactivity in the peripheral rim in the frontal or occipital view (Figure 12). Since the asymmetry of the peripheral vascular rim is the basis of the diagnosis, bilaterally symmetrical hematomas tend to escape detection [49].

The hematoma usually extends widely over the cerebral hemisphere, and the lateral view may show a diffuse increase in radioactivity but it is frequently normal and nonspecific. In a small number of cases with chronic subdural hematoma in the unusual location such as over the frontal or occipital lobe, however, the lateral view showing a vague but localized area of increased radioactivity provides a useful information for the correct placement of burr holes for evacuation (Figure 13).

It should be noted, however, that the crescent-shaped areas of increased radioactivity in the anterior or posterior view are not necessarily pathognomonic of the chronic

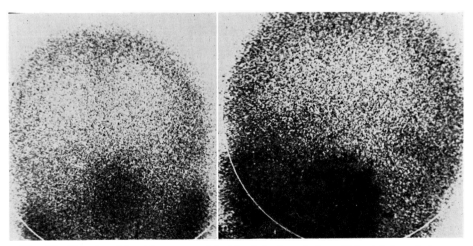

Fig. 12 Chronic subdural hematoma, left side. *Left:* frontal view; *Right:* left lateral view.

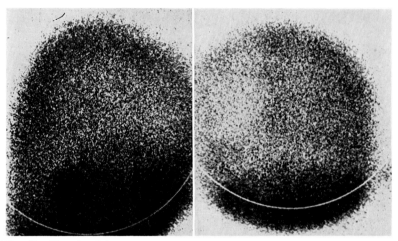

Fig. 13   Chronic subdural hematoma over the right occipital lobe. *Left:* right lateral
view; *Right:* occipital view.

subdural hematoma. A similar pattern may be observed in Paget's disease of the
skull, multiple carcinoma metastases to the skull, craniotomy defect, scalp trauma and
abrasions.   Cerebral ischemia resulting in the cortical infarction, some kinds of granulomatous pachymeningitis, and leukemic or tumor infiltrations of the meninges have been
reported to cause a crescentic shape of radioactivity. Even the common carotid
artery occlusion may show the asymmetry of peripheral vascular rim and simulate
the chronic subdural hematoma [60].

The site of accumulation of radioisotope in chronic subdural hematoma has not been
conclusively determined.   Kramer and Rovit [78], and Williams and Garcia-Bengochea
[161], have noted accumulation of chlormerodrin in the subdural fluid.   According to
Mealey and coworkers [99], however, abnormally increased radioactivity following administration of chlormerodrin in patients with chronic subdural hematoma is found
mainly in the hematoma membrane and not in the hematoma contents, and Gilson and
Gargano [41] have reported the experimental evidence that in dogs there is significantly
high uptake of radioactive mercury in the hematoma membrane than in the fluid.

Similarly using [203]Hg chlormerodrin as a tracer, Kobayashi [77] also reported that
the radioactivity in the hematoma membrane is higher than that in the hematoma
fluid.   Kobayashi further described the diffuse increase in the radioisotope uptake in the
hemisphere of the side of the lesion, and attributed this to the edema of the compressed
brain.

With ^{99m}Tc pertechnetate, several authors reported the relatively high radioactivity
again in the subdural membranes.   More recently, Morley and Langford [106] reported
four cases of subacute extradural hematomas with positive ^{99m}Tc pertechnetate brain
scans, and suggested that the nonspecific meningeal inflammatory reactions surrounding the hematoma are significant as the mechanism by which the abnormal scan is
caused.

Cowan and coworkers [23] suggested that the accuracy of diagnosis of subdural
hematomas is greater in cases which are older than 10 days, probably associating
with the development of the membrane.   This finding seems to support the hypo-

thesis of accumulation of radionuclide in the membrane than in the content of hematoma, and our results in several cases of subdural hematoma conform with this.

However, it may be redundant to decide whether it is the property of the hematoma membrane or accumulation of radionuclide within the hematoma content which produces the positive brain scan result. Both of the possibilities may be equally applicable, if it can be accepted that accumulation of radioisotope in the hematoma content is a result of membrane vascularity and permeability, as suggested by Morley and Langford [106]. Indeed, it may be expected that the main mechanism for the production of abnormal scan may be different among hematomas of various ages, and that the interval between the administration and scanning may possibly affect localization of the tracer.

Finally, it should be noted that the scanning may show positive results at least four to six weeks after surgery, when the repeat study is performed following the evacuation of hematoma in which the hematoma membrane has been left in place.

2.   Subdural Effusion in Infancy

The diagnostic value of brain scanning in post-meningitic or post-traumatic subdural effusion in infancy and childhood are not defined (Figure 64). David and coworkers [27] reported positive or suspicious results with ^{197}Hg chlormerodrin scanning in six children with subdural fluid collection, but the experience of Mishkin and Mealey [102], using either ^{99m}Tc pertechnetate or ^{197}Hg chlormerodrin, did not seem to be promising in 12 cases. Of nine patients with traumatic subdural effusion, three were scanned with ^{197}Hg chlormerodrin and all of them were negative. Nine cases scanned with ^{99m}Tc pertechnetate showed the abnormal foci, but the positive scan did not correlate with the clinical findings in all but one. In three cases of postmeningitic subdural fluid collection, scanning revealed the positive foci in all. In two of them with bilateral effusions, one scanned with ^{99m}Tc pertechnetate and one with ^{197}Hg chlormerodrin, abnormal radioactivity was found on one side only.

The poor scanning results observed in subdural effusion in infancy and childhood may be related to the absence or thinness of the capsular membranes. This seems to lend further support to the assumption that the positive scan in the adult subdural hematomas is due to the radioactivity in the membrane, which is much thicker and highly vascularized.

3.   Acute Subdural and Extradural Hematomas

In the typical cases of epidural hematoma, laceration of the middle meningeal artery usually results in a violent, rapidly fatal hemorrhage and the immediate surgery is indicated without preceding radiological studies. In such a fulminating case, brain scanning is not indicated, and we have no experience with acute cases.

When the epidural hematoma is of venous origin and the clinical course is protracted, as occasionally seen in the subacute epidural hematoma of parietal type or in the superior sagittal sinus hematoma, brain scanning has been performed and provided a useful information as to the atypical location of hematoma [106, 170].

Since the hematoma collects over the brain, its superficial crescent uptake is often difficult to differentiate from the abnormal radioactivity due to abrasion of the overlying scalp. The differentiation between the subdural and epidural location of hematoma is impossible and an arteriographic study is necessary for this purpose.

4. Intracerebral Hematoma and Cerebral Contusion

Frank intracerebral hematoma without accompanying extracerebral hematoma or cerebral contusion is rarely encountered after head injury. In cerebral contusion, the abnormal radioactive foci may be found in both frontal and lateral views. They are seen usually in the anterior temporal or the anterior frontal region, often bilaterally or on the side opposite the direct trauma. The abnormal foci usually resolve in five to 10 weeks on the follow-up scans. Scan images and their chronologic pattern in cerebral contusion may be similar to those of cerebral infarction, but the focus in contusion does not correlate with the territory of any cerebral artery.

Chapter IV

INFLAMMATORY DISEASES OF BRAIN AND MENINGES

The mechanism of radioisotope uptake in the inflammatory condition of the brain and meninges has not been fully known, and at present the definite conclusion can not be drawn concerning the ultimate role of brain scanning in the diagnosis of inflammatory diseases of the brain as a whole [2, 11, 34, 87, 113, 149].

1. *Brain Abscess and Granuloma*

Mishkin and Mealey [102] could detect 12 of 14 cases of abscess involving the cerebral hemisphere, but they missed both of two cerebellar abscess. Planiol [116] reported positive scan in 23 out of 24 cases of brain abscess. Our experience in scanning of brain abscess is limited, but we could detect all of five cases with proven cerebral abscess (Figure 14).

In addition, a case of granulomatous abscess in the subdural space believed to be one-year-old presented a positive result (Figure 15), but we missed one case of tuberculous granuloma in the frontal lobe, and another case of sarcoidosis in the hypothalamic region. Several other authors also reported relatively high detection accuracy in brain abscess, and we believe that the brain scanning is a sensitive method for early detection of supratentorial abscess.

Considering the ease and absolute safety of brain scanning, Teft and coworkers [149] concluded that the brain scanning could be used as a screening test for an early detection and better treatment of children with cyanotic heart disease. In their experience, brain scanning and electroencephalogram may show an abnormality earlier than angiography or air study presents the positive finding, and they reasoned that the scanning which represents the functional derangement in an involved area of the brain may possibly become positive before the contrast studies which show the anatomical abnormality tend to be abnormal.

In our experience as well as of others, no special characteristics were noted in the radioactive focus of brain abscess. Center of the focus may occasionally contain less radioactivity than the peripheral zone ("doughnut" sign or "halo" effect), but this indicates the non-homogeneity of the pathology and probably the cystic formation or necrosis, but is not necessarily pathognomonic of the brain abscess.

Scanning procedures provide a simple method of following the course of inflammatory process of the brain. Initially brain scan may be negative but it turns out to be positive as the disease process progresses to a frank cerebritis and abscess. Positive scan may return to normal after the prolonged antibiotic treatment for

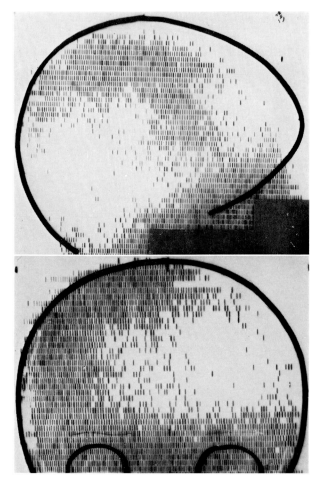

Fig. 14 Brain abscess. *Upper:* right lateral view; *Lower:* frontal view.

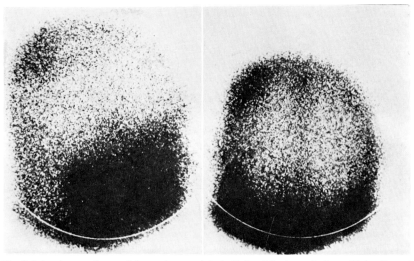

Fig. 15 Subdural granuloma, right parieto-occipital. *Left:* right lateral view; *Right:* frontal view.

presumed cerebritis, or after surgical evacuation of the ripe abscess.   The resolution of abnormal focus on the scan may correspond to the clinical improvements, but tends to persist long after clinical recovery [162].

2.   Meningitis and Encephalitis

DeLand and Wagner [29] described positive scans in a few cases of meningoence-phalitis.   In one case, the scan depicted the configuration of both lateral ventricles, and the autopsy proved the diagnosis of tuberculous ventriculitis.   In another case of a six-year-old boy, the area of increased radioactivity was noted to the right of the midline and over the left cerebral hemisphere in the anterior view, and in the region corresponding to the sylvian fissure in the left lateral view.   Purulent meningitis was confirmed by culture.

Balfour and coworkers [6] have reported a case of herpes simplex encephalitis which showed an abnormal uptake of radioisotope in brain scanning, and a few similar cases have since been reported by others.

We have so far experienced no positive scans in cases of meningitis or encephalitis, including tuberculous and mycotic meningitis proved by autopsy or cultures.

Chapter V

CEREBRAL INFARCTION

Differentiation of cerebral infarction from brain tumor remains to be a most important diagnostic problem. Because of the highly accurate localization of neural function in the territory of each cerebral artery, the causative vascular lesion may be suspected on the basis of a specific clinical syndrome. The most important syndromes produced by occlusion of certain cerebral arteries are summarized as follows [95] (Table 2).

1. Internal Carotid Artery

In autopsies on patients over 60 years without symptoms of cerebral vascular disease during life, an incidence of atherosclerotic occlusion of the internal carotid artery is about six per cent, and that of stenosis is much greater. In the patients with one or another symptoms of cerebral vascular disease, an incidence of significant carotid stenosis or occlusion found at angiography has been reported to be as high as 40 per cent. Men are affected twice as often as women, and the peak age incidence is 50–70 years.

Internal carotid artery supplies frontal, parietal and temporal operculum, caudate and lenticular nuclei, internal capsule, corona radiata as well as the retina and optic nerve. Clinically, it is impossible to distinguish the symptoms of internal carotid occlusion from those of stenosis. The signs and symptoms of internal carotid disease depend upon several factors;

1) the segment involved, especially whether it is above or below the origin of the ophthalmic artery,

2) the adequacy of available collateral circulation, and

3) rapidity of the occlusive process.

Clinically, occlusion or stenosis of the internal carotid artery may present as 1) recurrent episodes of reversible neurologic deficits (transient ischemic attacks or "TIAs"), 2) apoplectic form of onset, or 3) slowly progressive neurologic deficits.

In case with transient ischemic attacks, neurologic deficits subside completely within minutes to hours. Homolateral amaurosis fugax associated with the motor paresis or sensory disturbance on the side contralateral to the involved artery is pathognomonic of the internal carotid artery syndrome.

In case with an acute, apoplectic onset of disease, hemiplegia without previous episodes of carotid insufficiency is characteristic. This type of onset is seen in about 30–40 per cent of cases with carotid artery involvement and can not be definitely differentiated from the middle cerebral artery disease. Other conditions to be differentiated include the cerebral hemorrhage and embolism from the distant source.

Table 2 Clinical syndromes of occlusion of the cerebral arteries
(Modified from McHenry and Valsamiz[95])

Artery	Region of supply	Symptoms
Internal carotid	Frontal, parietal and temporal areas, caudate and lenticular nuclei, internal capsule and corona radiata, optic nerve and retina.	*Acute occlusion:* coma, aphasia (dominant side), contralateral hemiplegia, hemianesthesia, and homonymous hemianopia, ipsilateral blindness. *Chronic occlusion:* Transient attacks of hemiparesis, hemianesthesia, hemihypalgesia, monocular visual disturbance, etc.
Anterior cerebral	Anterior part of anterior limb of internal capsule, orbital surface and tip of frontal lobe, medial and parasagittal surface of brain up to parieto-occipital junction, anterior part of caudate nucleus.	Dementia, confusion, somnolence or coma, contralateral hemiplegia (severe in leg), and cortical sensory loss primarily affecting leg.
Middle cerebral	Convexity of cerebral hemisphere and its white matter, including lateral orbital frontal region and temporal tip. Perforating branches supply internal capsule, caudate and lenticular nuclei and anterior thalamus.	Syndrome similar to internal carotid occlusion except for absence of visual disturbance. *Partial infarction:* Partial contralateral motor and sensory disturbance, cortical sensory loss and weakness predominantly affecting arm. *Total infarction:* Coma, contralateral hemiplegia including the face, hemianesthesia, and homonymous hemianopia. Aphasia if dominant hemisphere is involved.
Posterior cerebral	Midbrain, including cerebral peduncles and third nerve, superior cerebellar peduncle, posterior part of thalamus, including lateral geniculate body, posterior part of internal capsule, base and posterior two-thirds of temporal lobe, splenium of corpus callosum, and medial surface of occipital lobe.	*Infarction involving the subthalamic nuclei:* Contralateral hemiballismus. *Infarction of thalamus and lateral geniculate body due to occlusion of thalamogeniculate branch:* Contralateral hemianopia and hemianesthesia. *Occlusion of calcarine branches:* Hemonymous superior quadrantanopia or hemianopia. *Occlusion of branch to basis pedunculi:* Ipsilateral third nerve palsy and contralateral hemiplegia with or without contralateral tremor.
Basilar	Structures of posterior fossa (pons, medulla, cerebellum) below bifurcation of basilar artery into posterior cerebral arteries.	Signs of abnormality involving third to twelfth cranial nerves in any combination, cerebellar disturbance, and long tract signs, especially corticospinal tract involvement.
Main trunk	Base and medial parts of tegmentum of midbrain and pons, including corticospinal tracts, corticobulbar tracts, oculomotor, trochlear, abducent and facial nerves, medial lemnisci.	Stupor or coma, hemiplegia or quadriplegia, dysarthria and dysphagia, pupillary abnormalities, paralysis of gaze or of ocular muscles and face, paresthesia and impaired vibratory and position sense.
Superior cerebellar	Lateral tegmentum of midbrain and upper pons, superior cerebellum.	Ipsilateral Horner's sign and cerebellar ataxia, contralateral loss of pain and temperature.
Posterior inferior cerebellar	Posterior and inferior parts of cerebellum, lateral tegmentum of medulla, including descending pupillodilator fibers, vestibular nuclei, descending nucleus and tract of trigeminal nerve, and glossopharyngeal and vagal nuclei, restiform body and dorsal spinocerebellar tract, lateral spinothalamic tract.	Ipsilateral Horner's signs, dizziness and nystagmus, ipsilateral loss of pain and temperature senses over face, dysphagia, dysphonia, ipsilateral cerebellar ataxia, contralateral loss of pain and temperature senses over arm, trunk and leg.

From 15 to 25 per cent of patients with internal carotid artery occlusion present the progressive neurologic deficits, and in this group of patients clinical picture may simulate that of brain tumor or other varieties of intracranial expanding lesions.

When the clinical picture is completed, contralateral hemiplegia or hemiparesis is seen in more than 75 per cent of cases. Other important symptoms are homonymous hemianopia, ipsilateral loss of vision, hemianesthesia and seizures, and aphasia when the dominant side is affected.

2. Middle Cerebral Artery

As a direct continuation of the internal carotid artery, the middle cerebral artery distributes to a major part of the convex lateral surface of cerebral hemisphere. From its origin, the middle cerebral artery turns laterally into the sylvian fissure, where it is encased by the frontal and temporal operculum. Arising from the proximal portion of the main stem of the middle cerebral artery, many perforating branches supply the putamen, globus pallidus, genu and posterior limb of the internal capsule.

Within the sylvian fissure, the middle cerebral artery divides into several branches which further travel in the sulci in the frontal, parietal, and superior surface of the temporal lobe. They are the ascending frontal, anterior and posterior temporal, posterior parietal and the angular arteries, which supply the insula, part of the orbital surface of the frontal lobe, inferior and the middle frontal gyri, most of precentral and postcentral gyri, superior and inferior parietal lobules, superior and middle temporal gyri and a part of the parietal lobe.

The middle cerebral artery as a whole supplies a much larger area than either the anterior cerebral or the posterior cerebral artery, carrying about 80 per cent of blood destined to the cerebral hemisphere.

The clinical symptom of occlusion of the middle cerebral artery or one or more of its branches varies widely, depending upon which branches are occluded and whether or not and how efficiently the collateral channels are available. Obstruction of the main trunk of the middle cerebral artery causes contralateral hemiplegia (most severe in the arm), hemisensory disturbance and homonymous hemianopia. Parietal lobe syndrome may occur, and when the dominant side is affected middle cerebral artery occlusion leads to an aphasia.

3. Anterior Cerebral Artery

The anterior cerebral artery proceeds anteriorly and medially from its origin from the internal carotid artery, crossing above the optic nerve and below the anterior perforate substance. From the horizontal segment of the artery, it gives off many perforating or ganglionic branches into the brain substance. Among them, the recurrent artery of Heubner or the medial striate artery is by far the largest, which arises from the anterior cerebral artery just proximal or just distal to the anterior communicating artery. Then it turns laterally over the anterior perforate substance and supplies a small portion of the orbital cortex of the frontal lobe and the anterior portion of the caudate nucleus as well as a part of the basal gnaglia and the anterior limb of the internal capsule.

The anterior cerebral artery distal to the anterior communicating artery, often named the pericallosal artery, runs around the genu of the corpus callosum and travels along the dorsal surface of the corpus callosum to the splenium. The pericallosal artery branches off the frontopolar artery, callosomarginal artery, and anterior, middle and posterior internal frontal arteries. Thus the anterior cerebral artery supplies the anterior part of the anterior limb of the internal capsule, orbital surface as well as the tip of the frontal lobe, medial and parasagittal surface of the cerebral hemisphere up to the parieto-occipital junction and the anterior part of the caudate nucleus.

As there exist variations of the proximal segment of the anterior cerebral artery in a high percentage of population, angiographic diagnosis of occlusion of the anterior cerebral artery may be difficult. In general, anterior cerebral infarction is rare by comparison. When it occurs, dementia, confusion or coma, contralateral hemiplegia (more severe in the leg) or monoplegia of the leg, and the cortical sensory loss primarily affecting the leg may be seen.

4. *Anterior Choroidal and Posterior Communicating Arteries*

The anterior choroidal artery supplies a portion of the posterior limb of the internal capsule as well as the globus pallidus and a part of the optic tract and the lateral geniculate body. The posterior communicating artery also branches off eight to 12 perforating branches supplying the hypothalamus and the neighbouring structures.

Although the occlusion of these arteries may occasionally produce respective clinical syndromes, its diagnosis does not seem to be possible on the basis of radioisotope scanning alone.

5. *Vertebral-Basilar Artery and Branches*

After arising from the subclavian artery, the vertebral artery ascends for a short distance in the posterior neck just medial to the scalenus anterior muscle, until it enters the foramen transversarium of the transverse process of the sixth cervical spine. Then the vertebral artery travels through the canal formed by the adjacent transverse foramina and ligaments up to the level of the second cervical spine, where it leaves the canal and runs around the posterior arch of the atlas and enters the skull through the foramen magnum. During its cervical course, the vertebral artery gives off twigs supplying the cervical nerves and ganglia, vertebrae, joints and muscles of the posterior neck.

Predilection site of the atherosclerotic occlusion of the vertebral artery is its origin from the subclavian artery. Congenital fibrous band and muscles attached to the cervical rib may compress the initial segment of the artery, and the osteoarthritic spur may compromise the lumen of the artery especially on turning the head.

Entering the skull, the vertebral arteries on both sides ascend medially and unite to form the midline basilar artery at the pontomedullary junction. Before uniting the vertebral artery gives off the anterior spinal ramus and the posterior inferior cerebellar artery.

The basilar artery ascends along the midline groove on the ventral surface of the pons up to the level of its junction with the brain stem. During its ascending course, the basilar artery branches off the superior cerebellar, anterior inferior cerebellar, auditory arteries and numerous perforating branches supplying the pons and the midbrain.

Blood carried by the vertebral-basilar system supplies fourth to twelfth cranial nerves, ascending and descending tracts of the pons and the medulla oblongata, cerebellum and the internal ear. Occlusion of the vertebral-basilar artery or its various branches often presents typical syndromes, but it is very rare to produce the positive radioisotope uptake on scanning.

6. *Posterior Inferior Cerebellar Artery*

The posterior inferior cerebellar artery supplies a wedge-shaped area of the medulla oblongata between its uppermost limit and the level of the gracile and cuneate nuclei. Infarction in the territory of the artery typically produces lateral medullary syndrome of Wallenberg, which includes vertigo, nausea, vomiting, nystagmus, dysphagia, ataxia,

Horner's syndrome and sensory disturbance of the face on the homolateral side and the contralateral hemisensory disturbance sparing the face. Although the lateral medullary syndrome is caused by the ischemia in the territory of the posterior inferior cerebellar artery, the causative lesion more often involves the vertebral artery than the posterior inferior cerebellar artery proper.

7. *Posterior Cerebral Artery*

The posterior cerebral artery usually is the terminal branch of the basilar artery, but in about 20–30 per cent of cases it originates from the internal carotid artery. The artery passes around the midbrain close to the free edge of the cerebellar tentorium, and reaches the inferomedial surface of the temporal lobe. Small perforating branches supply the cerebral peduncle, medial geniculate body and the colliculi. Thalamogeniculate branches nourish the pulvinar portion of the thalamus and the lateral geniculate body, and the medial and lateral posterior choroidal arteries terminate in the choroid plexus of the third ventricle, splenium of the corpus callosum and a portion of the thalamus.

Cortical branches of the posterior cerebral artery includes the anterior and posterior temporal, parieto-occipital and the calcarine arteries which supply the inferior surface of the temporal lobe, occipital lobe and a part of the parietal lobe.

Clinically, ischemia of the posterior cerebral artery leads to a homonymous visual field defect, and when occurred on the dominant side hemihypesthesia, dyslexia and loss of visual memory may be added to this. Occlusion of the thalamogeniculate branch of the posterior cerebral artery may cause the thalamic syndrome, in which loss of pain and temperature sensation is accompanied by a peculiar discomfort (anesthesia dolorosa).

It is to be remembered that, when the increased intracranial pressure leads to the herniation of the medial temporal lobe through the tentorial hiatus, compression on the posterior cerebral artery at the free edge of the tentorium may produce the ischemia and infarction of the occipital lobe with contralateral hemonymous hemianopia.

8. *Brain Scanning in Cerebral Vascular Occlusion*

The experience of brain scanning in cerebrovascular occlusive diseases has been reported by many authors, but the results differ widely for many reasons. Not all patients with occlusion of the cerebral arteries show abnormal scans, and the positivity seems to depend probably upon the size, nature, location of the cerebral lesion as well as the interval between the insult and the perfomance of scanning.

In some reports, only the carotid artery diseases are included whereas in others both the carotid and vertebral basilar diseases are reported together. It holds generally true that in the posterior fossa lesions the detection rate of brain scanning fails to reach that of the supratentorial lesions. It is especially true in the vascular occlusive lesions since the ischemia and infarction in the vertebrobasilar system of smaller size produce clear and discrete neurologic deficit than the lesion of the similar size does in the carotid artery territory. It follows therefore that the occlusive disease in the vertebrobasilar territory is much more difficult to detect by scanning. Practically, infarction in the posterior fossa can not be detected by scanning with few exceptions.

Furthermore, the true nature of the cerebral lesion is not verified pathologically in many cases diagnosed as cerebral vascular occlusion or as cerebral infarction. In some cases, the patient might have developed a frank infarction of the brain, whereas in others the vascular lesion caused temporary ischemia of the brain but the organic damage of the brain might well have been limited to the minimum because of efficiency of collateral circulation. Still in others cerebral hemorrhage might have been diagnosed as the occlusive disease. Therefore the composition of the reported series of patients is far from uniform and the wide range of difference in the detection rates of scanning may be expected.

Stebner and coworkers [141] correlated the brain scan and the autopsy finding in cerebral infarction. They found that the infarction in the cerebellum, basal ganglia and the occipital lobe could not be detected by scanning in their series. Eleven of 20 cases studied by both scanning and autopsy had all involved either frontal, parietal or temporal lobes.

Pattern and severity of the clinical symptoms apparently affect the accuracy of brain scanning in cerebral infarction. Transient ischemic attack does not usually produce the positive focus on scanning. Rhoton and coworkers [126], in reporting the large series of 50 cases of transient ischemic attacks as studied by ^{197}Hg and ^{203}Hg chlormerodrin scanning, noted the positive scan in none of them.

Sweet and coworkers [109, 144] noted that, when there was a persistent neurologic deficit due to cerebral infarction, arsenic brain scans were abnormal in 92 per cent of cases with severe, in 64 per cent with moderate, and in 83 per cent with mild deficits. In cases with temporary deficits, on the other hand, the degree of abnormality was only 47 per cent. In cases with transient ischemic attacks, a scan abnormality was seen in only two of 12 cases. Several other authors also have noted that the more severe the neurologic deficits, the more likely the brain scan will be positive.

Further, it has been stated that the positive scan in the patient suspected of harboring a cerebral infarction indicates a poor prognosis. Gutterman and Shenkin [46] reported 50 patients with completed stroke. Abnormal scan was obtained in 23 cases, and 22 of them had persistent neurologic deficits as compared to 20 of 27 patients with normal scans. Improvement in clinical symptoms was observed in 19 of 27 patients with normal scans, whereas in only seven of 23 cases with abnormal scan was there found a significant clinical recovery. Similarly, Glasgow and coworkers [42], Williams and Beiler [162] and several others also stressed the correlation between the abnormal brain scan and the prognosis as to the functional recovery in patient with cerebral infarction.

As to the etiology of cerebral vascular occlusive diseases, cerebral embolism has rarely produced the positive scan. Ojemann and coworkers [109], using positron emitting radioisotopes, reported 143 cases of cerebral vascular occlusion. Twenty-two of them showed transient ischemic attacks and the positive results were obtained in only four. Of 111 cases of cerebral thrombosis, 61 showed the positive scan. Eighty-six of those 111 cases presented the persistent neurologic deficits and in 25 cases symptoms were temporary. In the former group, positivity exceeded 60 per cent (53 of 86 cases), whereas in the latter group, only eight of 28 cases presented the positive scan (32 per cent). In contrast to the cerebral thrombosis, all of 10 cases of cerebral embolism failed to present the positive scan, irrespective of severity and duration of clinical symptoms.

In summary, it may be said that the positive scan is rarely obtained in cases of the transient ischemic attacks, embolic diseases or the infarction confined within the posterior fossa. Positive scan is less frequent in patients with mild neurologic deficits or symptom with good recovery than in cases with severe persistent deficits. Hemorrhagic infarction tends to show the positive scan more often than the anemic one [14]. It is obvious, therefore, that the results of brain scanning in cerebral vascular occlusion depend largely on the selection of cases referred to the scanning procedure.

Single, most important factor which determines the success of brain scanning in cerebral infarction is the interval between the onset of clinical symptoms and scanning. In the series of Mishkin and Mealey [102], brain scan showed an abnormal radioactive focus in 26 and it was normal in 16 when performed within one month after the occlusive episode. When scanning was carried out later, however, abnormality was found in only two of 12 studies.

Using ^{131}I RISA as a tracer, Planiol [116] repeated the brain scanning in 34 cases in which the initial study had been definitely abnormal. In all of them, repeat scanning performed two to eight weeks later showed that the abnormal radioactive focus had restored to normal.

Similarly but using [197]Hg or [203]Hg chlormerodrin, Rhoton and coworkers [127] reported 14 cases of cerebral infarction with definitely abnormal initial scan. In six cases, scanning was repeated within four weeks and the accumulation of radioisotope was decreased in one and increased in the other one. Repeat scanning was performed in four cases during the fourth to eighth week and the decrease in radioactivity was noted in two. At the eighth week and later, decrease was observed in six out of seven cases studied, and in three of them, the brain scan actually restored to normal.

With [197]Hg chlormerodrin, Yamamoto and Feindel [168] classified the contour brain scans of cerebral infarction as *negative*, less than 15 per cent differential uptake, and *positive*, more than 15 per cent difference. The time interval from the clinical onset to scanning was divided into six divisions. Angiographic findings were graded into five groups;

Group A:—demonstration of occluded cerebral arteries,

Group B:—indirect evidence of occlusion of branches of cerebral arteries, such as retrograde filling, slow filling or abnormal vascular area,

Group C:—marked stenosis of internal carotid artery without evidence of occlusion of cerebral arteries,

Group D:—occlusion of internal carotid artery in the neck with good collateral filling, and

Group E:—normal angiographic findings.

In group A, 32 out of 40 scans presented the positive results. In groups B and C, 29 out of 53 scans were positive and in groups D and E, only seven of 37 scans proved to be positive.

As to the interval from the onset to the scan, the positivities were 75 per cent within one day after the clinical onset, 46 per cent during two to seven days, 52 per cent at one to four weeks, 66 per cent at one to three months, 50 per cent at three to 12 months and 0 per cent in scans performed one year or more after the clinical onset.

Their results seemed to indicate that there is a close correlation between the angiographic findings and the positivity of scanning. On the other hand, the time interval between the clinical onset and the scanning in their series as a whole was not a factor in the occurrence of the positive scan.

They further compared the degree of differential uptake and the time interval between the onset and scanning. When the angiography demonstrated direct evidence of occluded cerebral arteries, the highest differential uptake was noted between the end of the first week and the third month, with the early scans tending to show a lower uptake. When the angiography showed only indirect signs of arterial occlusion, on the other hand, the uptakes were somewhat lower generally, suggesting less extensive cerebral damage.

Again using ^{197}Hg and ^{203}Hg chlormerodrin, Overton [113] reported the temporal changes in positivity in cerebral infarction. Brain scan was positive in 57 per cent during 0 to two weeks after the onset of clinical symptoms, in 83 per cent during three to four weeks, 38 per cent during five to 12 weeks and 0 per cent at 13th week or later.

With the positron emitting radioisotope ^{74}As, Ojemann and coworkers [109] achieved the positive scans in 15 of 20 cases of cerebral infarction within seven days after the clinical episode. During the second week and third to fourth week, the positivity remained essentially the same (eight of 11 cases and eight of 10 cases, respectively), but at the fifth week and later, it diminished acutely.

Molinari's result [104] with ^{99m}Tc pertechnetate also showed the similar trends, the positivity was highest during the second to fourth week, and sixth week or later, the scanning was almost invariably negative.

Thus, in general, cerebral infarcts may present a negative scan during the initial several days to one week after the clinical onset. Then there is an increasing ratio of positivity and during the second to third week, 70 to 80 per cent of cerebral softening will be detected by scanning. The abnormal accumulations of radioactivities then tend to decrease in the density, size and sharpness of the margins and most of them restore to normal after 60–80 days [42, 83, 113, 162]. However, a positive scan in cerebral infarction may rarely persist for several months to even one year; this is usually seen in exceptionally large, massive infarction.

Thus, serial scannings performed with an interval of several days to a week or two in between not only increase the detection rate of cerebral infarction but also they can frequently clarify the nature of the disease process. In many cases of cerebral infarction brain scanning provides more information than any of the other investigations such as electroencephalogram, pneumoencephalogram or even cerebral angiography. In these cases, there is actually damaged tissue of significant size but it often does not lead to the distortion of the vessels or the ventricles, and therefore it does not cause the deviation of these structures so as to produce significant angiographic or pneumographic abnormalities. Arteriography usually is an important diagnostic aid in demonstrating the site of vascular occlusion, but the recanalization or fragmentation and distal migration of the occluding thrombus or emboli does cause the negative angiograms in a significant number of cases.

In this connection, the recent paper of Rösler, Huber and Hesse [130] is very important and promising. Using a gamma-ray scintillation camera and ^{99m}Tc pertechnetate, they performed 83 brain scans in 72 patients of cerebral infarction. The patients were selected on the basis of clinical symptoms alone (Figures 16–19).

When the conventional scans were reviewed only 45 per cent of cases gave a positive delineation of the infarcts, with the best results of 80 per cent positivity obtained during the third week after insult.

In addition to the conventional scintigrams obtained 30 minutes or more after the administration of ^{99m}Tc pertechnetate (their step III study), however, they recorded

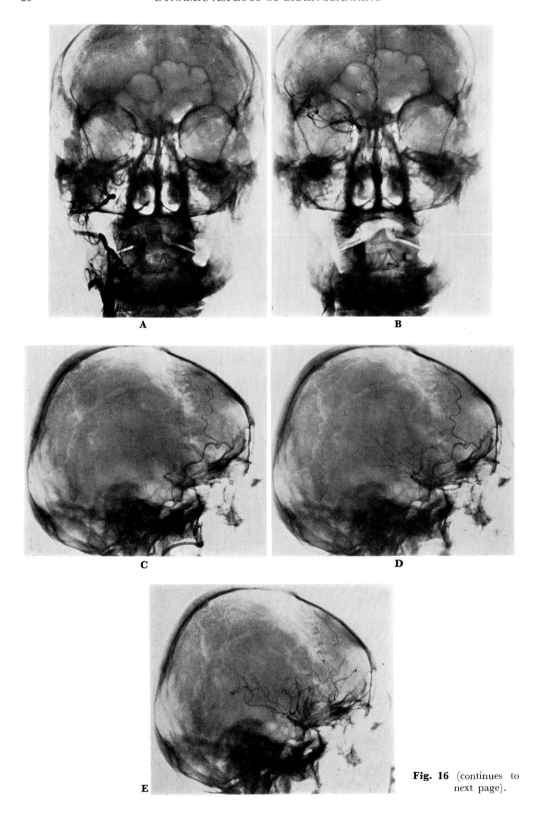

A   B

C   D

E

Fig. 16 (continues to next page).

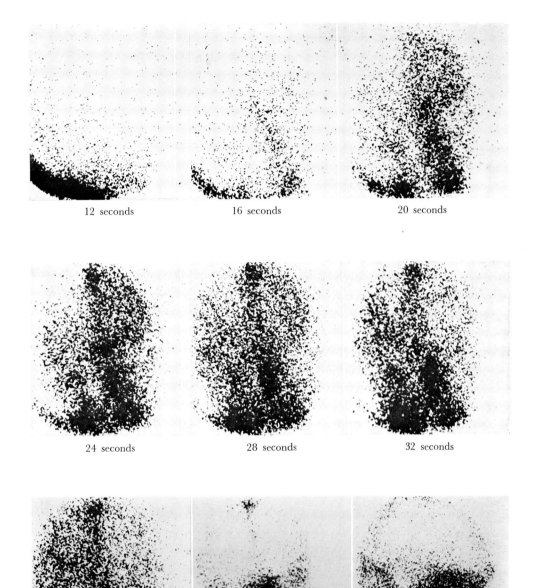

12 seconds   16 seconds   20 seconds

24 seconds   28 seconds   32 seconds

36 seconds   3 minutes   3 minutes

Fig. 16 A 78-year-old man with acute left hemiplegia. Angiography and scintigraphy a few days
after stroke. Angiography revealed right internal carotid artery occlusion in the neck.
Good collateral circulation from the external carotid artery through the ophthalmic
artery (**A** through **E**). Four-second exposure scintigrams in frontal view showed a delay
in the filling of the right hemisphere which showed only the arterial system when the
normal left hemisphere started to empty. In the conventional films taken three minutes
after administration of ^{99m}Tc pertechnetate, there is not yet an accumulation of
radioactivity in the infarcted focus.

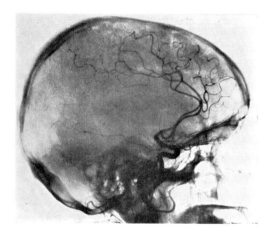

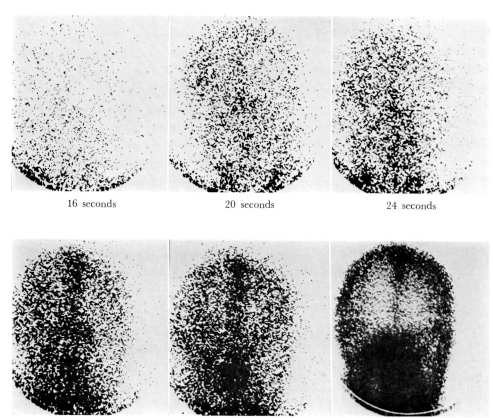

Fig. 17 A 47-year-old man with acute right hemiplegia and aphasia two days before examination. Angiography revealed an occlusion of the middle cerebral artery with collateral circulation via the leptomeningeal anastomoses. Frontal views of four-second exposure scintigrams revealed the occlusion of the middle cerebral artery, but the conventional films taken three minutes later failed to reveal the typical picture of infarction. The patient died later of pulmonary and renewed cerebral embolizations. At autopsy a large infarcted area was found in the temporal and precentral area and extending into the internal capsule. The age of the infarction was compatible with the initial attack of middle cerebral occlusion.

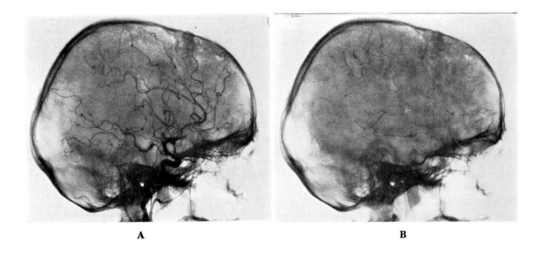

A   B

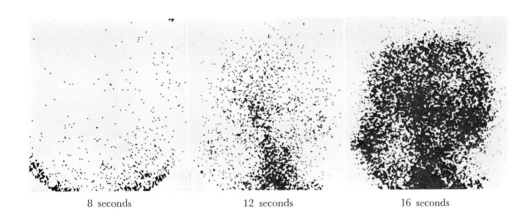

8 seconds   12 seconds   16 seconds

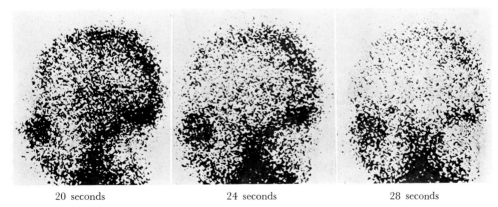

20 seconds   24 seconds   28 seconds

Fig. 18 (continues to next page).

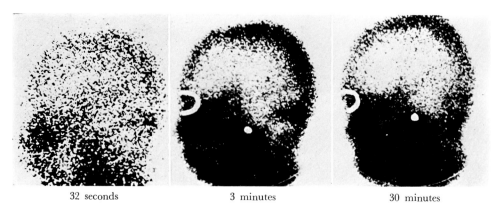

32 seconds   3 minutes   30 minutes

Fig. 18 A 32-year-old man with acute hemiplegia two days before examination. Angiography revealed the branch occlusion of the middle cerebral artery in the parietal region. Arteries in the ischemic area remained visible for a longer period. Four-second exposure scintigrams revealed the rather cool area in the parietal region, corresponding to the infarcted area. Around the cool area, a relatively hot ring is noted. In the conventional scintigrams, there is noted no typical infarcted area.

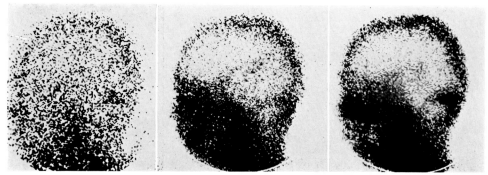

Fig. 19 The same case as in Fig. 18. Scintigraphy was repeated three weeks later. Radioactivity accumulation is noted in the angular region. (32 seconds, three minutes and 30 minutes after injection of ^{99m}Tc pertechnetate.)

also the serial scintigrams during the first circulation of the radionuclide through the cerebral vascular bed (radioangiography or step I study in their nomenclature), and the vascular scintigram (step II study).   For the purpose of step I study, eight serial films with four second exposure for each were obtained starting from the rapid injection of 10–15 mCi of ^{99m}Tc pertechnetate as a bolus into the antecubital vein. During serial scintiphotography, three phases were differentiated; in the *arterial phase* the large arteries in the neck and the main cerebral arterial trunks were visualized. Passage of radioisotope through the arterioles, capillaries, and venules was seen during the *parenchymatous stage*, and venous outflow during the *venous phase*.   Step II scintigrams were obtained three minutes after injection and they were believed to represent the distribution of the blood pool in the head and the brain.

When these serial studies were combined, a normal scan was obtained in no instance of 72 patients studied, although 18 studies were performed within six days and another 22 studies two months or more after the clinical onset.   The over-all detection rate was therefore increased to 100 per cent irrespective of the interval between the onset of clinical symptoms and performance of brain scanning.

Pathologic features in whole series of their cases were classified into four categories;

1) regionally increased accumulation of radioactivity as revealed in step II and step III studies (This was positive in 39 studies out of 83).

2) occlusion of or defect of cerebral arterial images, as observed in the arterial phase of step I study (This was most often seen, in 60 examinations out of 83).

3) and 4) dyssynchronization of the parenchymatous perfusion.

Phase dissociation was seen as the intensified accumulation of the radioisotope over the affected hemisphere in 3) and as reduced accumulation in 4).

Intensified focal perfusion in the parenchymatous phase associated with regional increase in radioactivity in the vascular and conventional scintigrams (Features 1 and 3 combined) was often seen during the second and third week after the onset. In the earlier stage or in the long standing lesions, occlusion or defect in the arterial phase and the reduced perfusion over the affected hemisphere were the predominant signs. Their results are quoted in Table 3.

Table 3   Results of brain scanning in 72 cases of cerebrovascular occlusive diseases
(Rösler, Huber and Hesse[130])

Interval between onset and examination	Number of examination	Radionuclide angiography negative	3 minutes scintigraphy positive	Conventional scintigraphy positive
<6 Days	18	0	5	7
7–13 Days	19	2	7	13
14–20 Days	9	1	6	7
21–60 Days	15	0	3	7
>60 Days	22	0	1	3
Total	83	3 (8%)	22 (27%)	37 (45%)

This detailed study clearly shows that the use of dynamic study does greatly increase the diagnostic accuracy of brain scanning in cerebral infarction. The precise location of occlusion or the degree of stenosis and the availability of collateral circulation can not be determined by this method, nevertheless, the detection rate of 100 per cent in 72 patients by Rösler, Huber and Hesse is quite excellent, particularly in view of the absolute safety of the scanning technic. The examinations provide additional criteria for the understanding of cerebrovascular insult as a disease which follows its own course.

The use of radionuclide transit curve study combined with photographic recording of radioangiography and vascular scintigraphy is expected to further increase the diagnostic accuracy in cerebral vascular occlusions. Recording the transit curve over each hemisphere, Yamamoto and Feindel [168] noted a time delay from the injection to cerebral peak on the affected side. In 29 cases with occlusive vascular disease and positive angiographic findings (Group 1, occlusion of cerebral arteries and Group 2, occlusion of the internal carotid artery in the neck with good cerebral collateral circulation) peak time on the pathologic side was delayed more than 0.6 second compared to the normal side. In Groups 3 and 4 with normal angiogram or where angiography was not done, the interval from the injection to the cerebral peak on the affected side was delayed and in 13 out of 22 cases the delay was more than 0.5 second.

9. *Mechanism of Positive Scan in Cerebral Infarction*

In connection with the temporal course of radioisotope uptake in cerebral infarction, the mechanism of positive scan has long been disputed. It might be supposed that the edematous tissue in and around the infarct collects the radioisotope, namely that the imparied barrier mechanism is the causative factor for selective accumulation of radioactivity in the ischemic focus.

Reporting the experience of sequential scanning in four cases of cerebral infarction, Rhoton [125] noted that the differential uptake at 3 hours postinjection was much higher than that obtained immediately after administration of ^{197}Hg or ^{203}Hg chlormero-drin. Waxman and coworkers [157] also found that the result of ^{203}Hg chlormerodrin brain scanning was much better at four hours after injection than earlier. Using this and other radionuclides, several other authors reported the similar results in sequential scanning. These progressive increase in differential uptake in cerebral infarcts may be considered to support the view that the main cause for radioisotope accumulation is the local breakdown of the barrier mechanism secondary to tissue anoxia.

When the brain tissue is rendered severely ischemic by arterial occlusion, however, there occurs a recognizable brain edema within several hours, and it often reaches the maximum in two to three days. Nevertheless, brain scanning performed within several days after the onset of clinical symptoms is often negative.

When the cerebral artery is occluded by thrombus or embolus, its perfusion area is rendered ischemic, and the size of the resultant infarct is determined by the availability of the collateral circulation. In case where the collateral circulation is efficient, the brain tissue may well escape persistent damage. When the collateral circulation is deficient because of the poor development of leptomeningeal anastomoses, anomalous configuration of the circle of Willis, aging process in the arterial wall or associated systemic hypotension, the central portion of the territory of the occluded artery becomes totally devoid of the circulating blood, and the radioisotope can reach there not directly from the circulating blood but only by diffusion from the border zone with decreased but still maintained perfusion. Accompanying edema, which elevates the tissue pressure, further compromises the circulation and increases the size of non-perfusion area. This might explain, to some extent at least, the low positivity of the brain scanning in the acute phase of cerebral infarction when it is accompanied by tissue edema.

Eventually, the ischemic tissue becomes infarcted and sometimes it is liquefied, and the reparative process involving the proliferation of glial cells is completed in six to eight weeks. At this stage or later, brain scan generally restores to normal. Thus, any of the impaired functions of the blood-brain-barrier, tissue anoxia and cell destruction, and reactive gliosis might not alone be responsible for the production of positive scan in cerebral infarction.

Severe ischemia with total shut-off of the circulation causes anemic infarction, whereas the hemorrhagic or red softening indicates that the circulation is still maintained by the collateral route or by lysis or distal migration of the occluding thrombus or embolus. This might explain the higher positivity of scanning in hemorrhagic infarction compared with the anemic one.

Histologically, reactive capillary proliferation in the infarcted tissue reaches the maximum degree during the third to fifth week after the insult and this coincides with the period when the positivity of scanning is highest. Molinari and coworkers [104], for this reason, considered that the capillary proliferation or the resultant increase in the tissue blood content represents the cause for focal accumulation of radioactivity. If the increased blood content is the sole factor in radioisotope accumulation, however, the focal radioactivity would be highest, and consequently the scintigraphic lesion most clear and vivid, shortly after administration of the tracer when its concentration in the blood is high. Actually this is not so, and the time course of radioisotope accumulation generally shows the progressive pattern and not the regressive one.

In the case of cerebral infarction illustrated in Figure 80, the scintigram taken shortly after intravenous injection of ^{99m}Tc pertechnetate revealed a cold central core surrounded by a zone of circular, hot band. Then the initial cold central portion became gradually hot and at the end of sequential studies 120 minutes after injection, the doughnut appearance noted in the initial phase was lost. When the time course of differential uptake in the central core was plotted, it showed a typical pattern of progressive impregnation.

In the peripheral zone, the situation was quite different; the uptake ratio remained stable or it rather decreased with time. In this particular case, preceding carotid angiography had demonstrated an avascular central area surrounded by a perifocal capillary blush in the right parieto-occipital region. Therefore, it seems reasonable to suppose that the situations were quite different in the two areas; in the peripheral zone of hyperemia, increased tissue blood volume might well be the main factor for the positive scan, whereas in the central core of frank infarction, impaired perfusion associated with the breakdown of the barrier mechanism may be responsible for the progressive increase in uptake. In this case, repeat scan three weeks later failed to disclose the peripheral zone of high radioactivity. Brain scan was equivocal in the early phase of sequential study, and later the focus as a whole demonstrated an ever increasing, homogeneous accumulation of radioactivity.

From these and other results, it seems that the mechanism of radioisotope accumulation in cerebral infarction is not single, but that loss of perfusion, breakdown of barrier mechanism, increased tissue blood volume due to proliferation of capillaries or the luxury perfusion, and possibly many other factors cause the complex pattern of uptake in various portions of the infarcted foci and at different ages of lesion.

Chapter VI

BRAIN SCANNING IN DISEASES OF SKULL

Many kinds of diseases of the skull bone, such as osteoid osteoma, fibrous dysplasia, hyperostosis in the acromegalics and healing surgical bone flap, may show up the positive brain scan. In these instances, it seems that the differential uptake of the radionuclide is seen in the area of reactive bone formation.

The brain scanning shows a positive uptake in the osteomyelitis of the skull (Figures 20 and 21). In this case, the inflammatory changes in the skull and the dura, namely

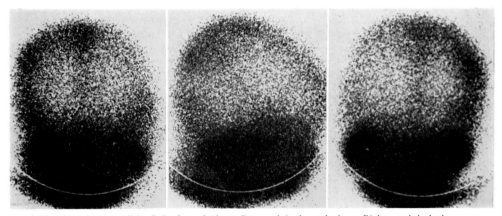

Fig. 20 Osteomyelitis. *Left:* frontal view; *Center:* right lateral view; *Right:* occipital view.

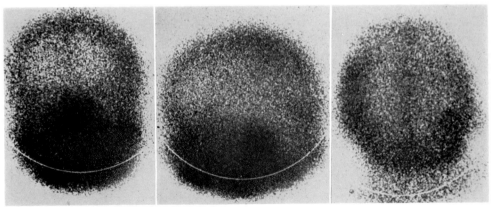

Fig. 21 Osteomyelitis. *Left:* frontal view; *Center:* left lateral view; *Right:* vertex view.

the proliferation of the blood vessels, formation of granulation tissue and an increased permeability of the involved vessels, play an important part in the radionuclide accumulation. Generally, such lesions of the bone tend to show more affinity for strontium than for the usual brain scanning agent. In questionable cases in routine brain scans, repeat strontium scanning and comparison with the plain skull films will confirm the location of the uptake.

The metastatic tumor of the skull is an another important group of diseases of the skull which show the radioactivity accumulation in a high percentage of cases (Figures 22 and 23).

Malignant tumors of the epipharynx often destroys the base of the skull and the cancer of the paranasal sinuses may erode the skull and invade intracranially. Such tumors, however, are often difficult to detect by scintigraphy because of their location near the skull base (Figure 24).

Other lesions which may produce bone changes in the skull base are the glomus jugulare tumors and chordomas, which may occasionally be detected by scanning of the head (Figure 109).

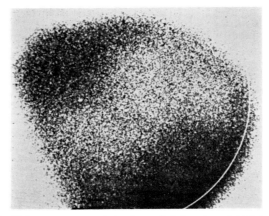

Fig. 22   Melanoma metastasis in the occipital region, right lateral view.

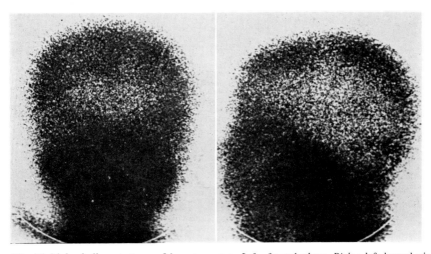

Fig. 23   Multiple skull metastases of breast cancer. *Left:* frontal view; *Right:* left lateral view.

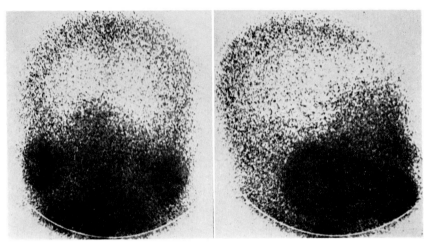

Fig. 24   Carcinoma of the frontal sinus. *Left:* frontal view; *Right:* right lateral view.

Almost any tumors which metastasize to the bone may metastasize to the skull. Primary sites of carcinoma metastasizing most often to the skull include the breast, prostate and the thyroid.   Carcinoma of the lung, kidney, gastrointestinal tract may occasionally involve the skull.   Skull metastases are often multiple, but may be solitary.   In such a metastatic tumor of the skull, main factor for the positive scan seems to be a differential uptake of radionuclide in the neoplastic tissue, and the new formation of the bone is of minor importance.

Other infrequent lesions of the skull which may be detected by scanning include dermoid and epidermoid tumors, eosinophilic granuloma and xanthoma, plasmacytoma, Hand-Schüller-Christian's disease and cavernous hemangioma of the skull (Figure 25).

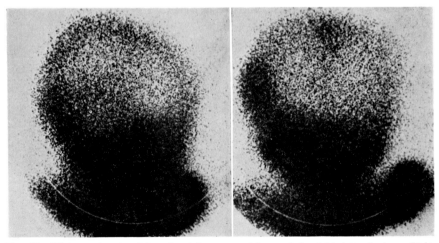

Fig. 25   Histiocytosis-x involving the right temporal bone. *Left:* right lateral view; *Right:* frontal view.

Chapter VII

CEREBRAL ANEURYSM AND ARTERIOVENOUS MALFORMATION

1. Cerebral Aneurysm

Positive radioisotopic imaging of the aneurysm *per se* belongs to an exceptional experience [8], apparently due to the small size of most of the aneurysms and their location at the base of the brain.

We have experienced a positive scan in a single case of giant aneurysms of both internal carotid arteries. Immediately after intravenous administration of ^{99m}Tc pertechnetate, frontal and lateral scintigrams revealed a sharp focus of increased radioactivity in the suprasellar region (Figure 26). Thereafter the uptake decreased rapidly and the repeat scintigram 10 minutes later and the conventional rectilinear scanning 30 minutes later were both entirely normal.

Since the radioactivity in the blood pooled in the aneurysmal sac is a sole mechanism for positive scan in aneurysms not associated with hemorrhage or infarction, the lesion is best depicted during the initial passage of the isotope bolus, and the rapid imaging with a scintillation camera is evidently preferable to conventional scanning.

Several authors have reported the results of brain scanning in subarachnoid hemorrhage due to ruptured cerebral aneurysm [21, 116, 144]. However, most of their positive scans were obtained in cases complicated with cerebral infarction, and therefore not specific to aneurysm. Although the positive scan in patient with subarachnoid

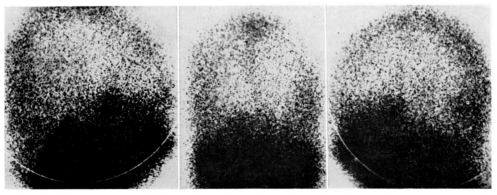

Fig. 26 Giant aneurysms of bilateral internal carotid arteries. *Left:* right lateral view; *Center:* frontal view; *Right:* left lateral view.

hemorrhage showing no lateralizing signs may be of some clinical value in deciding the side for the further arteriographic study, the infarction is not necessarily limited to the territory of the parent artery [24].

2. *Arteriovenous Anomaly*

Of 21 cases of arteriovenous anomalies studied by us in the past four years, 19 were cerebral arteriovenous malformations and two were racemose angiomas mainly involving the scalp. In no case were they associated with recent hemorrhage or seizures. Sequential ^{99m}Tc pertechnetate scintigraphy in these 21 cases showed definite abnormalities in all, including two patients whose lesions measured less than 2 cm in diameter (Figures 27, 28, 74, 75 and 76).

The maximum density of the lesion varied from case to case, but the focus was best shown always in the earliest phase of sequential studies. When the first stage scintigrams were exposed during the initial circulation of an isotope bolus through the lesion, not only the malformation itself but also the large vessels feeding and draining

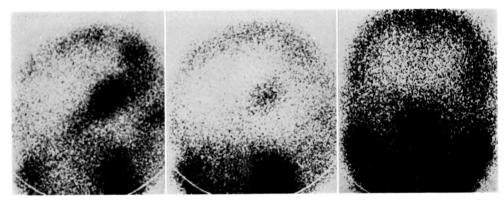

Fig. 27 Arteriovenous malformation in the left retrosylvian region. *Left:* immediately after; and *Center:* 10 minutes after administration of ^{99m}Tc pertechnetate. Left lateral view. *Right:* frontal view.

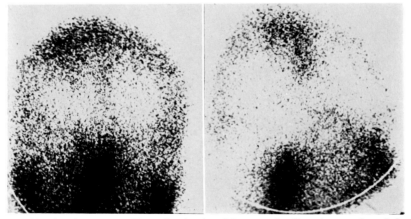

Fig. 28 Arteriovenous malformation in the right posterior frontal convexity. *Left:* frontal view; *Right:* right lateral view.

the anomalies could be demonstrated. Thereafter, the accumulation of radioactivity showed an acute decrease and the active focus tended to fade more or less rapidly. In at least five cases with smaller lesions, delayed scintigrams 30–60 minutes after injection was "equivocal" or practically "normal." In retrospect, therefore, the overall detection rate might have remained at 60–70 per cent, if the scintigrams were only obtained 30–60 minutes after injection and not earlier.

There are wide variations in the reported diagnostic accuracy of brain scanning in the arteriovenous anomaly, the detection rates being scattered between 15 per cent [86] and 100 per cent [165] (Table 4). Such discrepancies among the previous authors are

Table 4 Reported diagnostic accuracy of brain scanning in cerebral arteriovenous anomalies

Authors	Year	Radionuclide	Positive	Questionable	Negative	Total
Schlesinger et al. [139]	1962	^{131}I RISA	9	0	1	10
Overton et al. [113,114]	1965	^{197}Hg and ^{203}Hg Chlormerodrin	5	1	5	11
Planiol [117]	1966	^{131}I RISA	46	3	2	51
Ciric et al. [21]	1967	^{197}Hg Chlormerodrin and ^{99m}Tc Pertechnetate	10	3	6	19
Budabin [18]	1967	^{131}I RISA	18	0	6	24
		^{197}Hg Chlormerodrin	7	0	4	11
Witcofski et al. [165]	1967	^{99m}Tc Pertechnetate	14	0	0	14
Rasmussen et al. [124]	1970	"	6	3	2	11
Handa	1971	"	21	0	0	21

due, at least to some extent, to the radionuclide and instrumentation utilized, but the interval between the radioisotope administration and the examination evidently played the most important role [48]. Our results indicate that the optimum visualization with ^{99m}Tc pertechnetate is obtained immediately after administration. Schlesinger and coworkers [139], using ^{131}I RISA, successfully scanned nine of 10 cases, and they also found that the radioactive foci were best seen immediately after injection. Similar results with ^{131}I RISA was reported by Planiol [116], who detected 47 out of 57 cases, and 95 per cent of the positive scans were obtained in the early phase of serial studies.

As far as not being associated with recent hemorrhage or infarction, the main factor, if not the sole one, for the positive scan in arteriovenous anomaly, is the increased blood pool in the conglomeration of the dilated and elongated vessels in and around the lesion [18], and this apparently explains the higher positive scan results in the earliest phase of sequential studies.

Meningioma also is demonstrated best in the early phase of sequential scintigraphy, and after this, the focus loses its high radioactivity. The active focus in the meningioma is usually round to oval, denser and more sharply demarcated with clearer margin than in the arteriovenous anomaly. In the meningioma, moreover, the maximum uptake is observed somewhat later, the washout of radioisotope is not accelerated but rather delayed and the feeding vessels have not been visualized in radionuclide angiography.

Chapter VIII

NEOPLASMS

1. Meningioma

Meningiomas are the most common brain tumors as a single entity, and at the same time one of the most favorable kinds of lesion for brain scanning. Since they are essentially benign in their biological behavior and the permanent cure of the patient can be expected by a radical surgical removal, clinical significance of brain scanning for the purpose of their early detection cannot be overemphasized. Their frequency in the large reported series ranges from 13.4 per cent in all brain tumors as reported by Cushing and Eisenhardt [26], to 18.0 per cent of 6,000 cases of Zülch [171] or 19.2 per cent of 5,250 cases of Olivecrona [111].

Although the meningiomas may occur at any age, their incidence is greatest in the middle age and later. Since the meningiomas arise from the arachnoid villi [140], there exist several sites of predilection corresponding to the distribution of the arachnoid villi which later develop into the Pacchionian granulation.

They are arranged in order of frequency;

1) Meningiomas of the superior sagittal sinus, or parasagittal meningiomas. They are most common in the middle third of the superior sagittal sinus, less common in the anterior and rare in the posterior third (Figures 29, 30, 31 and 32).

2) Meningioma of the cerebral convexity. They are distributed over the whole convexity but the majority lie anterior to the rolandic fissure (Figure 77).

3) Meningioma of the sphenoid ridge and the sylvian fissure (Figure 33). They may be round but often flat like a plaque or carpet (*en plaque* type of meningioma).

4) Meningioma of the olfactory groove or the cribriform plate (Figures 34 and 35).

5) Meningiomas of the tuberculum sellae (suprasellar meningiomas or prechiasmal meningiomas), or of the planum sphenoidale (Figures 36 and 37).

6) Meningiomas of the tentorium (peritorcular meningiomas) (Figure 38). They grow either supratentorially, or infratentorially over the superior surface of the cerebellum, or both.

7) Meningiomas of the temporal fossa and Meckel's cave (Figure 39).

8) Meningiomas of the falx.

9) Meningiomas of the cerebello-pontine angle.

10) Meningiomas of the lateral ventricle.

11) Meningiomas of the clivus or craniospinal meningiomas.

12) Spinal meningiomas.

In addition,

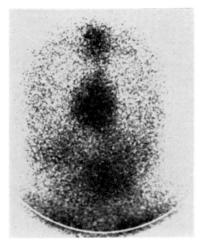

Fig. 29 Parasagittal meningioma attatched to the anterior
limit of the superior sagittal sinus. Frontal view.

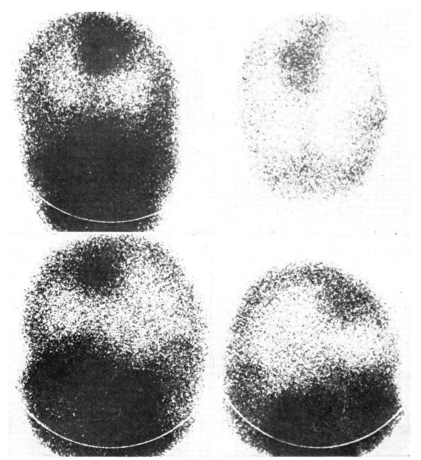

Fig. 30 Left parasagittal meningioma. *Upper left:* frontal; *Upper right:* vertex; *Lower left:* left lateral; *Lower right:* right lateral view.

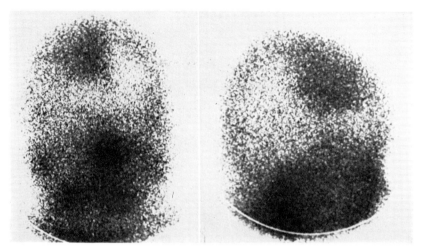

Fig. 31 Right parasagittal meningioma. *Left:* frontal view; *Right:* right lateral view.

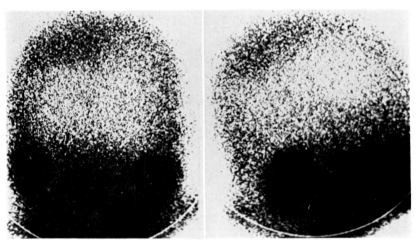

Fig. 32 Right parasagittal meningioma. *Left:* frontal view; *Right:* right lateral view.

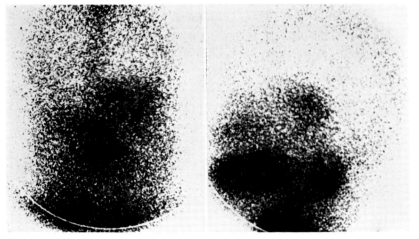

Fig. 33 Left sphenoid ridge meningioma. *Left:* frontal view; *Right:* left lateral view.

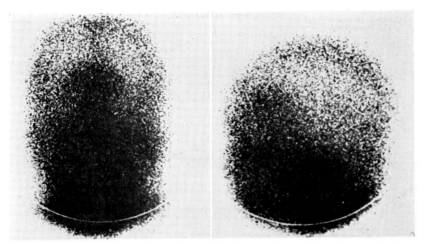

Fig. 34 Olfactory groove meningioma. *Left:* frontal view; *Right:* left lateral view.

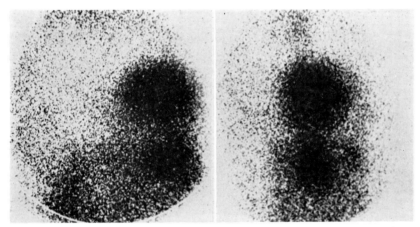

Fig. 35 Olfactory groove meningioma. *Left:* right lateral view; *Right:* frontal view.

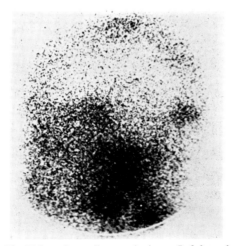

Fig. 36 Tuberculum sellae meningioma. Left lateral view.

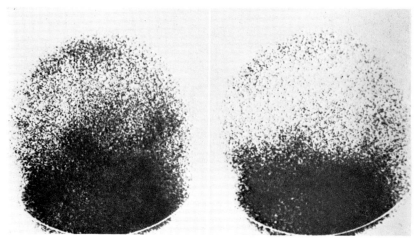

Fig. 37 Tuberculum sellae meningioma. *Left:* left lateral view immediately after administration of ⁹⁹ᵐTc pertechnetate; *Right:* left lateral view 10 minutes later.

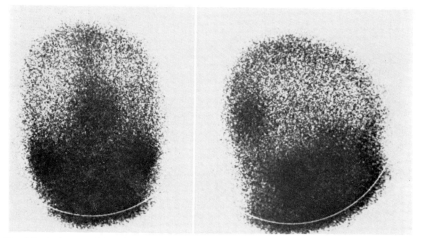

Fig. 38 Meningioma arising from the confluens. *Left:* occipital view; *Right:* right lateral view.

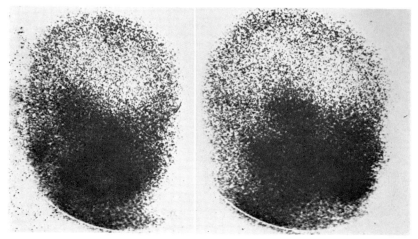

Fig. 39 Meningioma arising from the petrous dura. *Left:* frontal view; *Right:* right lateral view.

13) meningiomas may be multiple on rare occasions and they may be associated with acoustic nerve tumors or other neurinomas or neurofibromas in von Recklinghausen's disease.

The knowledge of the sites of predilection often provides a useful clue in predicting the type of lesion by scanning only; however, it should be noted that other kinds of tumors, either primary or secondary, can present the images quite similar to the meningioma both in their location and rounded configuration.

Diagnostic accuracy of meningioma by brain scanning is very high, and most authors reported the detection rates reaching or well exceeding the 90 per cent level [117, 159] (Table 5). The site of the tumor evidently has significant influence on the

Table 5 Detection accuracy of meningioma by scanning with various kinds of radionuclides

Authors	Radionuclide used	Total number of cases	Per cent positive
Paul and Morley [115]	RISA	37	81%
MaAfee and Taxdal [94]	RISA	13	100
Planiol [117]	RISA	241	93
Brinkman et al. [10]	Hg	13	77
Bucy & Ciric[16] [16]	Hg	15	93
Wang [155]	Hg	13	92
Wilcke [159]	Cu	73	96
Aronow [3]	As	112	84
Handa	Tc	32	94
Rasmussen et al. [124]	Tc	59	97

diagnostic accuracy, as revealed from the fact that the undetected meningiomas are usually located in the third ventricle, on the clivus, near the posterior lacerate foramen, over the cerebellar convexity, on both sides of the superior sagittal sinus [1], at the juguum [4], at the frontotemporal suture or at the temporal base. When the tumors near or at the base of the skull and in the posterior cranial fossa are excluded from the statistics, scanning scarcely fails to detect meningiomas.

Scan of a meningioma shows dense, discrete and homogeneous radioisotope concentration, shaped oval or round with sharp margin. When the sequential scintiscanning is performed, the meningioma appears immediately or shortly after the intravenous administration of ^{99m}Tc pertechnetate as a localized clear focus. After this, the focus loses its high radioactivity more or less rapidly, but the lesion generally remains distinct at the end of the serial studies covering 60–120 minutes after the injection (Figures 77 and 78). When such a characteristic picture is obtained in the predilection site of meningioma, prediction of the pathology is often possible. If the long history of clinical symptoms, and local bony changes on the plain skull x-rays are found in addition, the diagnosis of meningioma is highly accurate. Indeed, Planiol [116] reported that the pathologic diagnosis of meningioma was established on the basis of scanning in 72 per cent of her personal cases. The use of the first stage study in addition to the ordinary scanning is very useful for differentiation of meningioma from other pathologies, particularly from arteriovenous malformations, as shown later.

However, it should be borne in mind that the other tumors may possibly produce a round and dense focus of radioisotope uptake in the parasagittal and other locations typical for the meningiomas, and the meningioma, though rare, may show a delayed and progressive isotope accumulation and an irregular or plaque-like configuration.

Parasagittal meningioma and meningioma of the falx are diagnosed by brain scanning in almost 100 per cent of cases. Glioma of high grade malignancy may have a similar appearance, but the bulk of glioma is in the subcortical area, not related to the meninges, and often extends across the midline. In parasagittal meningioma, the focus lies adjacent to the midline of the convexity of the skull, and the medial border of radioactive focus is often straight in the frontal or posterior view, merging with the superior sagittal sinus uptake. Vertex view is very useful in displaying the anatomical relationship of the tumor with the sagittal sinus. Usually, the tumor is oval in shape but occasionally it is flat like a carpet (Figure 32). Falx meningioma often lies on both sides of the falx cerebri so that the radioactive focus is found in the midline.

Meningioma arising from the olfactory groove reaches a large size before the patient comes to the examination, so that the brain scanning is a very useful screening method of examination (Figures 34 and 35). Meningiomas of the tuberculum sellae, or suprasellar meningiomas, on the other hand, encroach upon the optic nerves and chiasm in early stage while they are still small in size (Figures 36 and 37). Because of the small dimension and the basal location of the tumor, they may prove difficult to detect by brain scanning. In the anterior view, the tumor may be obscured by the high background activity in the nasal mucosa and facial muscles, unless the head is well-flexed. In the lateral view, a localized increase in radioactivity may be mistaken for activity in the sphenoparietal sinus and arteries and veins in the sylvian fissure.

Meningioma at the temporal base or of the middle third of the sphenoid wing may also escape detection. Some of deep temporal meningiomas are barely visible at the first early examination, however, they become clear and detectable during the subsequent runs [116].

The posterior fossa meningiomas are generally best detected in the conventional or angled posterior view.

In our experience of more than 30 cases of meningiomas, brain scanning failed to reveal the lesion in two cases, one case of small tuberculum sellae meningioma and the other one case of an *en plaque* type meningioma at the base of the middle fossa. Angiographic and histologic studies have shown that no exact parallelism exists between the density of radioactivity in the focus and the vascularity of the tumor.

2. Cavernous Angioma of Brain

Cavernous angioma of the brain, or the cavernoma, is rare and we have experienced brain scanning of a large tumor of this kind only twice, both of which were positive. The tumor showed a well-defined, round to oval and dense concentration of radioactivity early in the sequential scanning, and the focus tended to fade with time.

The pattern of scintigrams therefore are quite similar to that of the meningioma, and their differentiation seems to be impossible from the scintigraphic point of view (Figure 40).

3. Metastatic Tumor

Intracranial metastatic tumors account for 3.4 per cent in the 5,250 cases of Olivecrona's series [111] and 3.2 per cent in Chshing's series [25]. The above figures

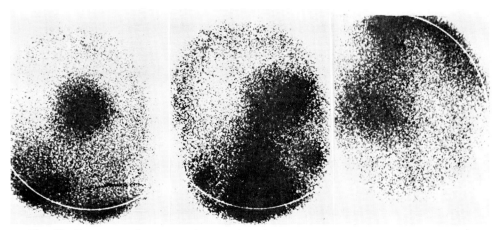

Fig. 40 Cavernoma of cavernous sinus. *Left:* Left lateral; *Center:* frontal; *Right:* vertex view.

are derived from the neurosurgical clinics, and it may be argued that they are unduly low because the cases in which cerebral metastases are obvious would not have been accepted for surgical treatment. On the pathological point of view, Courville [22] estimated that an incidence of 20.5 per cent of all intracranial tumors is probably as close an approximation as can be obtained, and Störtebecker [142] also quoted figures ranging from 13.5 per cent to 37 per cent.

In recent yearr, an incidence of metastatic brain tumors has been steadily increasing in the neurosurgical clinic, and now its diagnosis and treatment have become a very important task for the neurosurgeon. In our personal experience, an incidence of around 20 per cent of all intracranial tumors seems to be an acceptable estimate.

The great majority of intracranial metastases are carcinomas, and sarcomas are rare. As to the primary sites of the carcinomas, lung is the most common source accounting for approximately 50 per cent of all metastatic carcinomas, followed by carcinomas of the breast, cancer of the gastrointestinal tract and renal tumors (Table 6).

Metastases to the brain may become manifest months or even years after the first recognition of the primary neoplasm. Some sixty per cent of cases, however, show the symptoms referable to the brain before the appearance of symptoms due to the primary tumor [72], and in about 10 per cent of them the primary tumor can not be found at the time of examination for cerebral metastasis. Since the metastatic brain

Table 6 Primary sites of metastatic carcinomas in
the brain (Kahn[72])

Primary sites	Number of cases	Per cent
Lung	36	48 %
Breast	13	17.3
GI tract	7	9.3
Thyroid	2	2.6
Kidney	2	2.6
Uterus	2	2.6
Others	3	4.0
Unknown	10	13.3
Total	75	

tumor occurs most frequently in patients 40–60 years of age, the brian tumor cases in this age group should always be checked carefully for the possible secondary nature of the lesion.

Accuracy of detection of metastatic tumors has always been complicated by the fact that the small metastatic nodules, usually with the diameter of 2 cm or smaller, are not rare, in which resolution capacity of the equipment may not allow for detection even when they are located in the favorable sites for scanning. When they are accompanied by a peritumoral zone of edema, however, edematous brain may be detected as an area of relatively poor radioactivity in the earliest phase, or as a blurred focus with progressive radionuclide accumulation in the later phase of sequential scintiscanning. Accordingly, sequential studies including the serial first stage scintigram during the initial passage of the injected radionuclide is important for improving the detection accuracy (Figure 82).

Reported incidence of multiple metastatic deposits ranges widely, but it has been generally agreed that the secondary tumors of the brain are most often multiple [137]. Since the evidence of multiplicity is an important factor against the surgical treatment, all efforts should be paid for detecting the multiple lesions in brain scanning of the elderly patients.

Two independent radioactive foci in locations far from each other, one in the right cerebral hemisphere and the other in the left or one supratentorial lesion and the other one in the posterior cranial fossa, for example, most probably indicate the metastatic nature of the pathologies. Metastatic cerebral abscess may present a scan indistinguishable from multiple metastatic tumors [101], but we have not experienced such a case.

Separate but closely located foci, however, are not necessarily indicative of the metastatic nature of the lesions. Gliomas with central necrosis, hemorrhage or cystic formation may occasionally show the increased radioactivities in two or more separate locations, simulating the scan in multiple metastatic deposits.

Another fact to be remembered is that the positive brain scan in patient with malignant neoplasm elsewhere in the body does not always indicate the metastatic nature of the cerebral disease [122, 123]. We have experienced a case of astrocytoma developed years after treatment for lung cancer, and similar experiences of association of primary intracranial neoplasms and malignancies elsewhere have been reported. Cerebral vascular accidents comprise another more important group which is more apt to be associated with the extracerebral malignancies.

Metastatic carcinoma may take the form of diffuse dissemination of nodules in the meninges—the so-called carcinomatous meningitis or meningeal carcinosis. Multiple cranial nerve palsies including blindness, headache and face pain, nuchal rigidity and progressive dementia or impaired consciousness have been observed with or without symptoms and signs referable to the increased intracranial pressure. The cerebrospinal fluid which is high in protein content and low in sugar level may suggest the inflammatory process, and the diagnosis may prove very difficult. Brain scanning in such a case of diffuse meningeal dissemination does not help the diagnosis.

Evaluation of the results of brain scanning in metastatic tumors is made more difficult by the fact that the histologic control is often lacking, since a significant percentage of patients are discharged without confirmation of diagnosis by surgery or autopsy.

From a survey of the reported series and from our experience, however, it appears certain that the brain scanning achieves the detection accuracy of 80–90 per cent or even higher in the confirmed cases [110, 117, 128]. Although the diagnostic accuracy falls to 50 per cent level when the posterior cranial fossa metastases are considered separately [101], metastases are fortunately most commonly found subcortically in the cerebral hemisphere and particularly in the territory of the middle cerebral artery, the site most favorable for radioisotopic localization. Thus, excluding the meningeal carcinomatosis, the early detection of the metastatic tumor seems to be one of the best uses of brain scanning as a screening procedure, and we consider it reasonable to perform brain scanning in every patient harboring the neoplasm elsewhere in the body which can metastasize to the brain.

When small, metastatic nodules tend to be circumscribed and round. This may give a scan with round areas of increased radioisotopic uptake having rather discrete margins (Figure 41). When the metastatic nodules are surrounded by the perifocal brain edema, margin of the radioactive focus tends to become more blurred, and the size of the scintigraphic lesion appears often larger than the anatomic boundaries of the tumor (Figures 42, 43, 44 and 45).

The radioisotopic accumulation in the edematous brain may be responsible for the trends of progressive accumulation of radioactivities, which frequently characterizes time course of sequential scintigraphic studies. However, this is not always true, and the metastatic tumor may present a scan image of regressive course of radioisotope accumulation. In fact, we have experienced several cases of metastatic carcinomas which showed a clear, round focus with high radioactivity shortly after administration of radionuclide, and the radioactivity thereafter decreased rapidly, the picture not quite unlike that of meningioma (Figure 84). In all those cases, angiography demonstrated the discrete tumor vessels and the diagnosis was confirmed at operation.

As the metastases grow large, the central portion of the tumor may become necrotic. Brain scan discloses the central core of decreased uptake surrounded by a zone of increased radioactivity. While the scan images are unique, they are not necessarily pathognomonic of the metastases ("Halo" effect or "doughnut" sign in brain scanning).

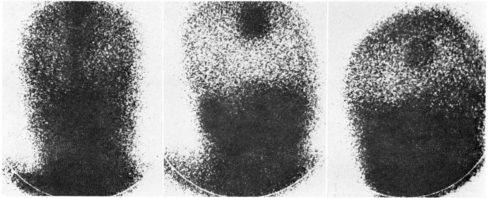

Fig. 41 Metastatic carcinoma in the left parasagittal region. *Left:* Frontal view immediately after administration of ^{99m}Tc pertechnetate; *Center:* frontal view 120 minutes later; *Right:* left lateral view 120 minutes later.

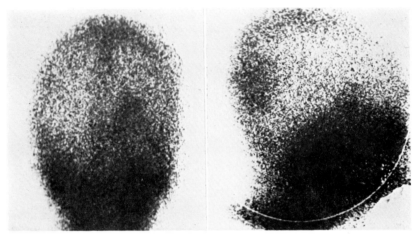

Fig. 42 Metastatic carcinoma (primary site breast) in the right occipital pole. *Left:* occipital view; *Right:* right lateral view.

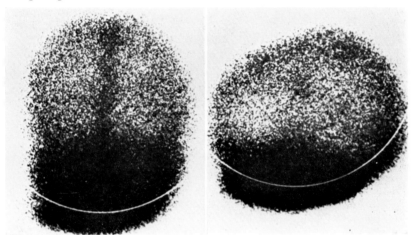

Fig. 43 Metastatic carcinoma in the left suprasylvian region. *Left:* frontal view; *Right:* left lateral view.

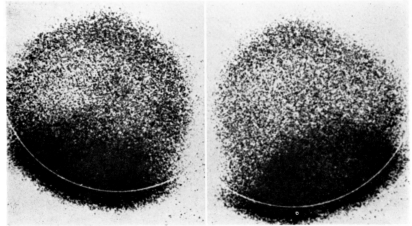

Fig. 44 Metastasis of chorion epithelioma in the left retrosylvian region. *Left:* left lateral view; *Right:* right lateral view.

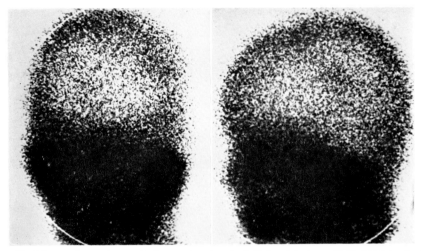

Fig. 45 Metastatic carcinoma (primary site; lung). *Left*, frontal view; *Right*, left lateral view.

High accumulation of ^{131}I RISA in metastatic carcinoma of the thyroid gland, or selective uptake of labeled chloroquine analogue in melanomas [7, 9] has been reported, but the nature of the primary lesion does not seem to play any significant role in the characteristics of the radioactive foci as far as the ^{99m}Tc pertechnetate brain scanning is concerned.

4. Glioblastoma

Glioblastoma is by far the most common brain tumor in the adult. It comprises 15–25 per cent of all intracranial tumors, and approximately 50 per cent of supratentorial gliomas are glioblastoma (Figures 46–49).

Glioblastoma is a highly malignant, rapidly growing, invasive and often highly vascular tumor, and calcification is rarely found. It may occur in any portion of the brain, but the occipital lobe tends to be spared for unknown reasons. It usually occurs in the subcortical white matter of the cerebral hemisphere and often invades the hemispheres bilaterally.

Glioblastoma can be detected by brain scanning very accurately, the diagnostic accuracy exceeding 90 per cent in most of the reported series (Mishkin and Mealey [102], 96 per cent; Ojemann [110], 95 per cent; Planiol [116], 93.5 per cent). In a few cases with initial negative or equivocal scans, repeat scanning several weeks to a few months later often presents the definitely abnormal accumulation of radioisotopes. According to Planiol [116], fairly differentiated type or "isomorphic" type of glioblastoma has less permeability to the labeled compounds than the more anaplastic forms and the false negative scan is obtained more often in the former group.

In the brain scan of glioblastoma, the focus shows more or less progressive accumulation of radioisotopes (Figure 81). When ^{99m}Tc pertechnetate is used as a tracer, the radioactive focus is not uncommonly ill-defined in the beginning, but it becomes more and more clear with the passage of time and the best image usually is obtained 30–60 minutes after administration. It is irregularly configurated, the density of accumulation of radioactivity is variable, but the margin of the focus is relatively distinct.

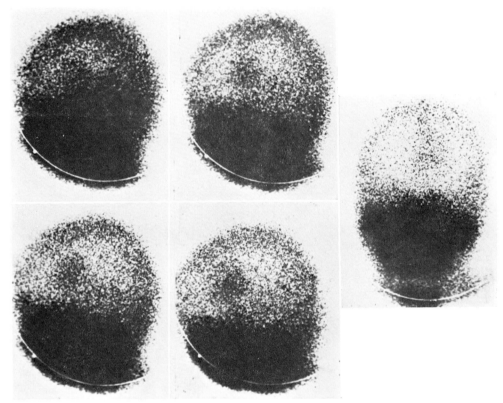

Fig. 46 Glioblastoma multiforme. *Upper left:* immediately after; *Upper right:* 15 minutes after; *Lower left:* 45 minutes after; *Lower right:* 60 minutes after administration of ^{99m}Tc pertechnetate.Left lateral views. *Right:* Frontal view.

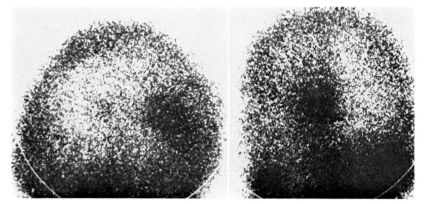

Fig. 47 Glioblastoma multiforme in the right frontal pole. *Left:* right lateral view; *Right:* frontal view.

Rapid growth of glioblastoma is represented in the necrosis of central portion of the tumor. This feature is faithfully reproduced on the brain scan as a halo of increased radioactivity surrounding the central core of low background activity ("halo" effect or "doughnut" sign). This is, however, not necessarily pathognomonic of the glioblastoma (Figure 87).

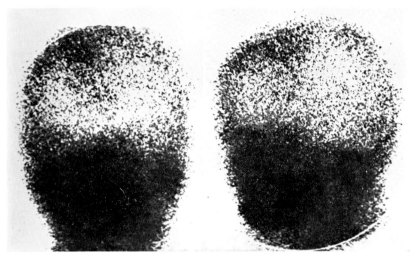

Fig. 48 Glioblastoma multiforme. *Left:* frontal view; *Right:* left lateral view.

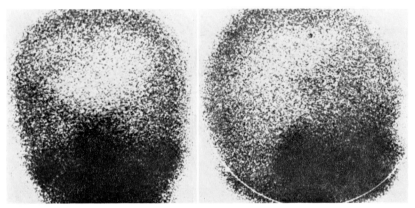

Fig. 49 Glioblastoma multiforme. *Left:* frontal view; *Right:* right lateral view.

In most cases of glioblastoma multiforme, the displacement of cerebral structures is so pronounced that the detection of a mass by air study or angiography is easy. Occasionally, however, it causes minimal displacement of ventricles and vessels in spite of extensive invasiveness.

This is particularly true of glioblastoma involving the corpus callosum, which is reported to occur in 35 per cent of autopsied cases [68, 169]. This type of lesion often proves to be difficult to localize by angiography, but it presents the peculiar "butterfly" configuration in the frontal or occipital view, and occasionally in the vertex view of the brain scan. Bilaterally expanded falx meningioma may produce somewhat similar findings, but the dense, round and sharply demarcated radioactivity aids in differentiation in most cases.

5. *Astrocytoma of Cerebrum*

Astrocytoma of the cerebrum is almost always infiltrative, slowly progressive, and calcification is found in approximately 10 to 20 per cent of cases. Although cerebellar astrocytomas are commonly cystic tumor with a mural nodule, cystic astrocytomas of the cerebrum are rare. The incidence of astrocytoma in all intracranial tumors ranges 6.4 per cent in 6,000 cases of Zülch's series [171], to 9.8 per cent or 10.5 per cent in Chshing's series [25] and Kahn's series [72], respectively.

Astrocytomas of the cerebrum occur in much the same age group and location as glioblastomas, furthermore, it is not rare to find a glioma in which varying degrees of anaplasias are found in different portions within the tumor. Hence, the histologic diagnosis from a piece of specimen, especially obtained by a needle biopsy, may be misleading. These facts make the overall detection rate of brain scanning less reliable.

Using ^{131}I RISA, Planiol [116] detected 57 of 101 astrocytomas (57 per cent positivity), in 38 brain scanning was negative and in 8 it was equivocal. It is not clear whether this report includes cerebellar astrocytoma or not. Mishkin and Mealey [102] reported somewhat better results, namely 78 per cent positivity, and our experience also shows the similar detection rate.

Brinkman [11] studied 29 astrocytomas, 24 of them were classified as grade 2, and 5 as grade 1. In the former group, 19 cases presented a positive scan (79 per cent) but in the latter, none was detected. Reviewing the literature, therefore, cerebral astrocytomas seem to be detectable in around 60 per cent of cases.

The appearances of the scan in astrocytoma are not specific (Figure 50). The uptake is noted usually deep within the cerebral hemisphere, its shape is irregular and the margin is not discrete. Degree of radionuclide accumulation is usually less than that of more malignant glioblastoma, but occasionally very high radioactivity with discrete margin may be found (Figure 58).

When the sequential imaging is performed, the astrocytoma shows a progressive accumulation of radioactivity (Figure 79). Initial scan shortly after administration of radionuclide is often negative, or shows only blurred focus. With passage of time, the focus becomes more and more distinct and the scan of best quality usually is achieved 45–60 minutes after administration of ^{99m}Tc pertechnetate.

6. *Oligodendroglioma*

Oligodendroglioma is a relatively uncommon tumor involving the cerebral hemisphere

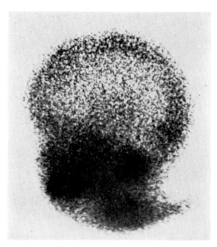

Fig. 50 Astrocytoma in the deep central portion. Left lateral view.

of the adult, its peak incidence being in the fifth decade. It is slowly progressive, biologically benign but infiltrative, and it tends to occur in the subcortical white matter and most often in the frontal lobe.

Grossly the tumor is most often solid and avascular with a fairly discrete margin and often shows calcifications visible on the skull films. The scan image shows no features which aid in the differentiation of oligodendroglioma from cerebral astrocytoma (Figure 51).

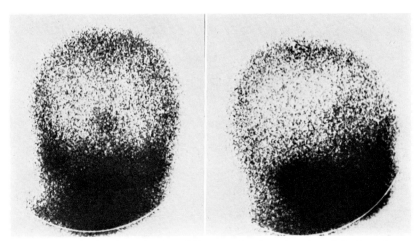

Fig. 51 Oligodendroglioma in the midline anterior frontal region. *Left:* frontal view; *Right:* right lateral view.

We have experienced two exceptional cases of oligodendroglioma with unusual hypervascularity noted on the carotid angiogram and at operation. In each case brain scanning revealed a circumscribed, distinct accumulation of radioactivity immediately after administration of ^{99m}Tc pertechnetate, which decreased rapidly in the course of sequential studies, the images not quite unlike those of meningioma (Figure 85).

7. *Ependymoma*

Ependymoma is a tumor of children and young adults which most commonly occurs in the fourth ventricle but may arise from the lateral ventricle. Rarely it may not be related to the ventricle, especially in infancy and early childhood.

The scan of cerebral ependymoma is not characteristic, the radioactivity is often uneven and has irregular outline. Its deep location within the ventricles is noted easily with three dimensional views.

Meningioma and choroid plexus papilloma may be found in the lateral ventricles, but they can be differentiated from ependymoma because of their uniform and more intense uptake of radioactivity. Astrocytoma or oligodendroglioma arising near the ventricles can not be differentiated from ependymoma (Figure 52).

Ependymoma in the fourth ventricle may be missed because of high radioactivity in the normal midline vascular channel such as the occipital sinus.

8. *Pituitary Adenoma and Craniopharyngioma*

Pituitary adenoma comprises 8.0 per cent in Zülch's 6,000 cases of all intracranial

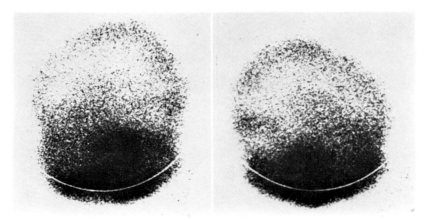

Fig. 52: Ependymoma. *Left:* left lateral view; *Right:* right lateral view.

tumors [171] and 8.5 per cent in Olivecrona's series of 5,250 cases [111]. Cushing [25] reported much higher incidence of 17.8 per cent, which is evidently due to his particular interest in this disorder and resultant case selection.

Although pituitary adenoma is one of the most common intracranial tumors, it can not be easily detected by scanning technic. Intrasellar adenoma, either chromophobe or eosinophilic, has never produced a positive scan in our experience; even in the chromophobe adenoma with large parasellar or suprasellar extension, the detection rate remained at around 50 per cent level.

The differential uptake of radioisotope does not seem to be too low to permit the external detection of pituitary adenoma, and the low diagnostic accuracy is mostly due to the anatomical factors.

First of all, endocrine and visual disturbances appear early while the tumor is still not large enough. Its basal location makes external detection difficult because of high background radioactivity in the muscles and nasal mucosa. Relatively large distance between the lesion and the external detector places the tumor out of the focal plane of collimator, no matter from which direction the scanning is performed.

When a large suprasellar pituitary adenoma shows a positive scan, lateral view demonstrates a globoid area of increased radioactivity in the region of the sella turcica. In the frontal view, the focus lies in the midline adjacent to the base of the skull but tends to be more ill-defined than in the lateral view (Figure 53).

The incidence of craniopharyngioma in the large reported series is 2.5 per cent in Zülch's series [171] or 1.7 per cent in Olivecrona's series [111]. The peak of incidence occurs between the ages 13 and 23 [171], and in childhood and adolescence cranio-pharyngiomas are the most common tumors in the chiasmal region.

Even when the tumor is large, craniopharyngioma does not seem to take up the radioisotope in sufficient amounts to be detected, and we have successfully visualized only one third of cases, in all of them the tumors located in the supra- and intrasellar region and they were very large in size (Figure 54).

Most authors have described that the craniopharyngiomas are difficult to detect be-cause of the presence of normal radioactivity in the structures surrounding this area. However, James and coworkers [71] recently reported that of 13 patients with histologically proven craniopharyngiomas they found the positive scans in 12.

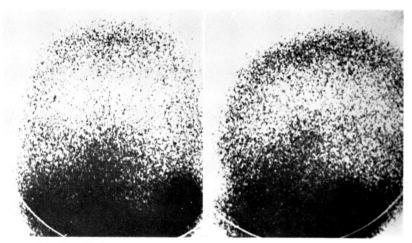

Fig. 53: Pituitary adenoma. *Left:* frontal view; *Right:* left lateral view.

When visualized by scanning, the lesion is best seen in the frontal view at the base of the brain and almost in the midline. In the lateral view, it lies in the suprasellar region, and it is least commonly detected in the occipital view or vertex view.

Craniopharyngioma can not be differentiated from the suprasellar extension of the pituitary adenoma or other suprasellar tumors on the basis of scanning alone.

The differential diagnosis of increased radioactivity in the sellar and suprasellar region includes suprasellar extension of the chromophobe adenoma of the pituitary, optic nerve glioma, planum sphenoidale meningioma or tuberculum sellae meningioma, meningioma of the medial third of the sphenoid ridge, large aneurysm of the cerebral arteries and, less commonly, solitary metastasis of carcinoma in this region and chordoma.

Skull x-rays provide sufficient information in the majority of cases. Hyperostotic changes associated with dense and homogeneous radioactivity in the brain scan is characteristic of meningioma. In pituitary adenoma, expansion of the sella turcica without calcification is usually found, and skull films shows in 80 per cent of

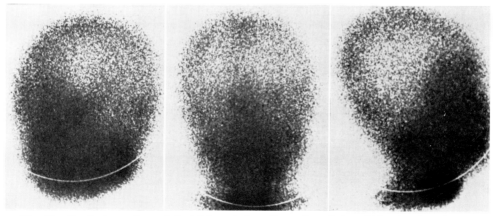

Fig. 54 Craniopharyngioma. *Left:* left lateral view; *Center:* frontal view; *Right:* right lateral view.

craniopharyngiomas calcification of the tumor. The calcification and a typical changes in the sella turcica help greatly to distinguish craniopharyngioma from pituitary adenoma. Glioma of the optic nerve is almost never calcified and often causes unilateral enlargement of the optic canal. Aneurysm of the cerebral artery, when large enough, may cause the positive scan, occasionally shows linear calcification of the aneurysmal sac and metastatic lesions are usually multiple, they do not calcify, and they are rare in the characteristic location of craniopharyngioma.

9. *Acoustic Neurinoma and Other Cerebellopontine Angle Tumors*

Tumors of the cerebellopontine angle account for 7 to 10 per cent of all brain tumors [171], and more than 90 per cent involve the eighth cranial nerve. Eighty per cent of them are neurinomas, seven per cent meningiomas and five per cent epidermoid tumors. Thus the acoustic neurinomas comprise 7.6 per cent in all intracranial tumors in 6,000 cases of Zülch's series [171], or 8.0 per cent of cases of Olivercona's series [111]. They are limited almost always to the adult, and occur often bilaterally in cases of von Recklinghausen's disease.

Although they locate in the posterior cranial fossa, they are detected by scanning technic in 70–80 per cent of cases. Mishkin and Mealey [102] reported 78 per cent positive results and the only two tumors missed were the tumors which occurred as the smaller one of bilateral tumors, and were not demonstrated by other x-ray technics.

Better result was reported by DeLand and Wagner [28]. Using ^{99m}Tc pertechnetate and a scintillation scanner, they successfully detected 12 of 14 cases (86 per cent positivity). Retrograde brachial arteriography was positive or suggestive in four of eight cases. Pneumoencephalography showed the lesion in three of five cases and positive contrast cisternography was successful in two of three cases examined. Accordingly, at least in this series, the accuracy of brain scanning seems to exceed that of other diagnostic procedures.

Acoustic neurinoma arises from the perineural tisue, probably the Schwann's cells of the cochlear nerve as it traverses the pia mater. This accounts for the site of origin of the tumor at the medial end of the internal acoustic meatus.

As the tumor enlarges, lateral extension is limited by the petrous bone, and inferior extension by a ledge of the occipital bone. Thus the tumor tends to expand posteriorly and medially.

When visualized by scanning technic, the lesions lie anterior to the sigmoid sinus, and when they are large they overlie the sinus. In the occipital view which is often crucial for detection of acoustic neurinoma, the internal auditory meatus is projected below the transverse sinus and the lesions appear to lie adjacent to and below the transverse sinus. Usually the abnormal radioactivity is round and discrete (Figures 55 and 56).

In cases of acoustic neurinomas, skull films almost invariably show erosion of the medial portion of the internal auditory meatus. The combination of the x-ray changes and the typical scan images along with the clinical symptoms of cerebellopontine angle mass allows the pathological diagnosis of acoustic neurinoma, though the meningioma in the cerebellopontine angle may show similar findings. Chordoma, epidermoid tumor and rarely glioma may occur in the cerebellopontine angle, but we have no experience of scanning in these tumors.

Recently more and more smaller tumors have been diagnosed and successfully

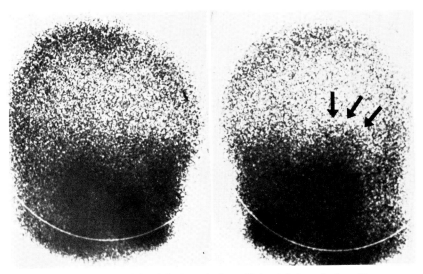

Fig. 55 Acoustic neurinoma. *Left:* right lateral view; *Right:* left lateral view. Tumor was on the left side.

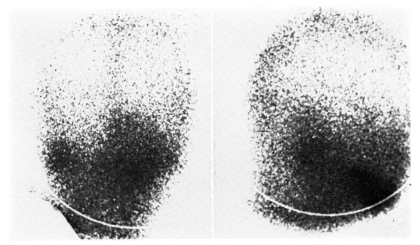

Fig. 56 Acoustic neurinoma on the right side. *Left:* occipital view; *Right:* right lateral view.

removed by surgery, preserving the function of the seventh and occasionally also eighth nerves. Such a small tumor, particularly the intracanalicular one, undoubtedly is the best candidate for surgery, but they can not be detected by scanning technics, and other diagnostic procedures such as the refined otologic tests and positive contrast cisternography are often necessary.

10. *Tumor of the Thalamus and Basal Ganglia*

Thalamic tumors are not common, they form about one per cent of all supratentorial tumors in the series of McKissock and Paine [96], and of Potts and Taveras [118]. Surgical resection or biopsy of these tumors may be dangerous and the radiotherapy and shunt operation are performed following the radiological localization. The tumors are grouped as tumors of the thalamus and basal ganglia since the pathologic diagnosis is lacking in most cases. Cheek and Taveras [20] obtained histologic confirmation in 24 of their 51 cases, 10 were astrocytomas, 11 glioblastomas, two were mixed oligodendroglioma and astrocytoma and one was an angiomatous malformation. In the cases of Tovi and coworkers [150], glioblastomas were more common. Twelve out of 22 cases were glioblastomas, six were astrocytomas and the rest of cases were two ependymomas and one each of oligodendroglioma and vascular malformation.

The thalamic tumors occur more often in young persons than in elderly individuals, and both sexes are affected equally. Duration of symptoms from the onset to admission varies widely, ranging from several days to years in the reported series, but a short history is more common.

Symptoms are nonspecific. Headache and vomiting are found in most patients, followed in frequency by failure of vision, mental changes, apathy and motor weakness or sensory disturbance. Main objective signs include papilledema, unequal pupils, abnormal pupillary reactions, visual field defects, facial paresis and ataxia. Thus the most common signs and symptoms are those referable to the raised intracranial pressure and the thalamic symdrome is rarely found in patients with thalamic tumors. Pupillary abnormalities are of great clinical significance. Thus, a fairly short history of increased intracranial pressure and the presence of hemiparesis, sensory disturbance, motor incoordination and pupillary abnormalities in the relatively young individual strongly suggest the tumor in this region, however, neuroradiologic examinations are indispensable for the accurate diagnosis.

Pneumoencephalography or ventriculography is the method of choice for diagnosis and localization of the thalamic tumor, but the patients clinically suspected of harboring a supratentorial tumor, especially when there are lateralizing signs, may usually be first investigated by carotid angiography, and in fact the thalamic tumors are most often looked over by this examination.

Vertebral angiography is more informative, but not all these tumors will be diagnosed with this method, particularly when the tumors are still small, and the false negative angiogram may delay the study by air encephalography or ventriculography.

Brain scanning often helps localizing the tumor in the thalamus and the basal ganglia. Lawrie [82] reported an area of increased radioactivity in the region of the thalamus in all of four cases, Castelli and coworkers [19] observed positive scans in approximately 50 per cent of midline and basal ganglia tumors and our results were essentially consonant with theirs.

In our experience lateral view is most useful and the frontal, occipital or vertex view rarely presents the positive scan. Radioactive foci are found deeply in the central portion of the brain, and are usually round to oval, blurred, with indistinct margin and the differential uptake is not high. In a few cases the uptake was so weak that the conventional scintigram was diagnosed negative, but the map and profile films demonstrated the lesion. Time course of uptake was variable, in some cases the focus appeared soon after administration of ^{99m}Tc pertechnetate, whereas in the other cases the best picture was obtained 30–60 minutes after injection. In the former group and when the tumor was small, it could not be differentiated from the uptake of the choroid plexus.

Figure 57 illustrates a lady presented with papilledema, bitemporal hemianopia and apathy. Carotid and vertebral angiographies revealed symmetric dilatation of the lateral ventricles, but the tumor could not be localized.

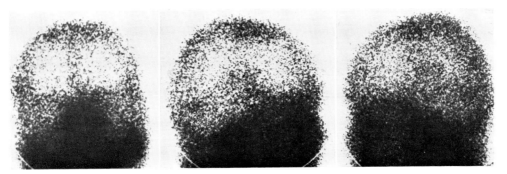

Fig. 57 Thalamic tumor, histology unknown. *Left:* frontal view; *Center:* right lateral view; *Right:* left lateral view.

Lateral view of the scintigram disclosed positive uptake in the central region but the frontal view was non-remarkable. Later, thalamic tumor obstructing the third ventricle was confirmed by iothalamate ventriculography. Bitemporal hemianopia in this case seems to have been caused by compression of the optic chiasm by the dilated third ventricle.

11. Choroid Plexus Papilloma

Choroid plexus papillomas are rare tumor of the brain occurring with an incidence of approximately 0.5 per cent of intracranial neoplasms in adults [25, 171] and 3.0 per cent to 5.0 per cent of brain tumors in children [81, 90].

Recently, Rovit and coworkers [136] collected 234 cases from the literature and added their own 11 cases. Of these 245 cases, 105 patients or 43 per cent, occurred in one of the lateral ventricles, 26 (10 per cent) in the third ventricle and 95 cases (39 per cent) in the fourth ventricle. In 3.7 per cent tumors are multiple. Preferential site of origin differed markedly between adults and children; the majority of the choroid plexus papillomas in children arose in the lateral ventricle, whereas in the adult tumors in the fourth ventricle predominated.

The majority of the choroid plexus papillomas occur within the first decade of life and are invariably associated with communicating hydrocephalus, and the inadequate bubble studies have been performed and the benign lesion missed in numerous cases.

Because of the rich vascularity of the tumor as well as the known accumulation of ^{99m}Tc pertechnetate in the choroid plexus [89, 164], one might expect that the ^{99m}Tc pertechnetate brain scanning would reveal a high degree of radioisotope uptake in cases with choroid plexus papillomas. Practically, however, there are only few reports regarding the brain scanning of this type of intracranial tumor. One reason for paucity of the reports, as has been suggested by Rovit and coworkers [136] may be that the scanning procedure has not been used widely for study of children with hydrocephalus.

12. Optic Pathway Glioma

Optic pathway gliomas primarily involve the children, and they can occur sporadically but often they are associated with von Recklinghausen's neurofibromatosis. The reports of positive brain scan in this disorder are few, and we have experienced only one case of positive result in brain scanning. In this case of a child with a huge astrocytoma which originated from the optic nerve but later involved the hypothalamus extensively, brain scan revealed a very marked concentration of radioisotope, as shown in Figure 58.

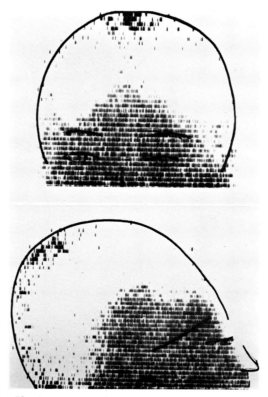

Fig. 58 Astrocytoma of the optic nerves and hypothalamus.

13. *Epidermoid and Dermoid Tumors*

Epidermoid and dermoid tumors are rare tumors of congenital or embryonic origin, and account for 1.9–0.7 per cent of all intracranial tumors. Their sites of pre-dilection are cerebellopontine angle, chiasmal region, longitudinal fissure and within the ventricle, but we have detected none of three cases encountered.

14. *Sarcoma*

Sarcomas of the brain account for 2.7 per cent in 6,000 cases of all intracranial tumors in Zülch's series [171], or 0.7 per cent in Cushing's series [25]. Kernohan and Uihlein [74] reported a somewhat higher incidence of three per cent, but they still belong to a rare variety of brain tumors.

We have experienced five cases of sarcomas, three of which were fibrosarcoma and two were reticulum cell sarcoma.

The brain scanning showed a definitely abnormal uptake in each of them (Figures 59 and 60). The focus showed an area of dense accumulation of radioactivity with a clear margin in three, and in the remaining two cases radioactivity was less pronounced and the focus was blurred. In one case of reticulum cell sarcoma with a central necrosis, a so-called "doughnut" sign was found in that the central area of relatively low radioactivity was surrounded by a peripheral ring of higher radioactivity (Figure 60). Thus the scan images are nonspecific and the pathological diagnosis does not seem to be possible by scanning procedure alone.

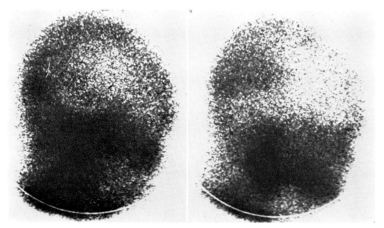

Fig. 59 Fibrosarcoma in the right occipital region. *Left:* right lateral view, immediately after administration of ^{99m}Tc pertechnetate; *Right:* 75 minutes later.

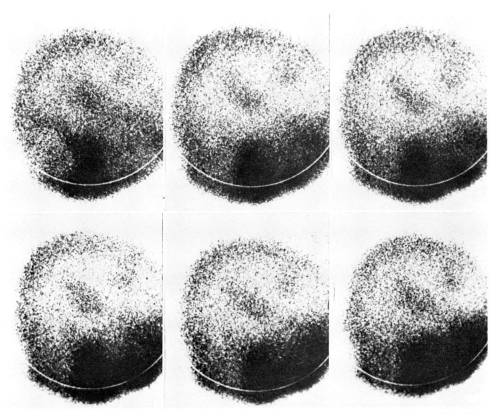

Fig. 60 Sarcoma. *Upper left:* Immediately after; *Upper center:* 15 minutes; *Upper right:* 30 minutes; *Lower left:* 45 minutes; *Lower center:* 60 minutes; and *Lower right:* 75 minutes after administration of ^{99m}Tc pertechnetate. Right lateral view.

15. Detection of Recurrent Tumors

Early detection of recurrence of tumor poses an important but often difficult problem. Many intracranial tumors, especially gliomas, can not be removed totally by surgery, and the palliation by partial removal or often biopsy alone and decompression by resection of the silent lobe or removal of the bone flap is all that can be done for the patient. Although they are often effective, postoperative radiotherapy and chemotherapy at the present status do not eradicate the tumor and the recurrence is inevitable.

When the decompression has been done, occurrence of symptoms and signs of increased intracranial pressure, such as headache, vomiting, visual disturbance and papilledema, is delayed to appear when the tumor regrows. If the secondary optic atrophy has been present, papilledema does not develop in the face of markedly increased intracranial pressure. Because of the preexisting deficits due either primarily to the neoplasm or secondarily to the preceding surgery, evaluation of neurologic and mental manifestations is rendered more difficult with recurrence of tumors.

Interpretation of radiologic examinations is also interfered with for several reasons. Preceding operations, particularly lobectomy, result in dislocation and distortion of configuration of the cerebral vessels and ventricles, and the mass effect of recurrent tumor often fails to cause typical changes on angiograms or pneumograms. In the presence of a recurrent tumor, lateral shift of the pineal calcification, anterior cerebral artery or the internal cerebral vein may be entirely lacking, and in fact those midline structures occasionally show the negative shift toward the side of the tumor. Air-filling of subarachnoid space is usually poor over the involved hemisphere, and the deformation of the ventricles may be secondary not to the recurrent tumor but to the previous operation. In our experience, contrast-filling of tumor stain or neoplastic vessels tends to be poor on angiograms obtained after decompression or irradiation. Electroencephalogram also does not help so much in early recognition of recurrence.

Radioactive brain scanning, on the other hand, does demonstrate the lesion itself, and it is expected to be superior to other indirect radiologic diagnostic methods for the localization of recurrence. It is a safe and not-unpleasant procedure and it can be repeatedly scheduled on an out-patient basis. Thus it has been our policy to follow up the patients in whom the recurrence of tumor is to be expected at various intervals by serial scanning. Interval varies according to the clinical state of the patients, but usually ranges from two to three months at the early post-operative period to six months or more later on. When any change in the clinical condition is noted, scanning is performed immediately. Further radiologic examinations—angiography or pneumography—are performed when the serial scanning demonstrates any suggestive changes of recurrence.

A case of glioblastoma multiforme in the left frontotemporal region is illustrated in Figure 61. Since March 1967, this 42-year-old school teacher had experienced several attacks of generalized convulsive seizures. When seen for the first time in March 1969, physical and neurological examinations disclosed no abnormalities and the eye grounds were normal. Spinal tap revealed a clear, colorless cerebrospinal fluid containing 52 mg/dl of protein and 82 mg/dl of sugar, the pressure was 185 mm of water. Brain scanning with ^{99m}Tc pertechnetate disclosed an abnormal collection of radioactivity in the left anterior temporal lobe (Figure 61, left), which showed a progressive course of accumulation on sequential studies. A diagnosis of left anterior temporal tumor was

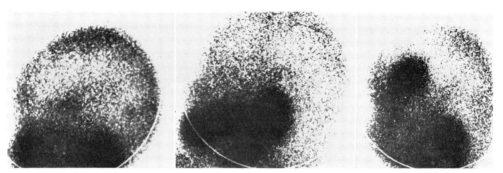

Fig. 61 Follow-up scans in a case of glioblastoma in the left frontotemporal region. *Left:* before operation; *Center:* after operation and irradiation; *Right:* recurrent tumor.

proved by angiography.

At operation, the tumor was found in the anterior portion of the left temporal lobe infiltrating deeply into the insula. Anterior temporal lobectomy was followed by postoperative irradiation with 6,000 r of ^{60}Co. Histologically, the specimen seemed to represent astrocytoma grade II. When discharged, the patient showed the right upper quadrantic homonymous field defect and a slight degree of amnestic aphasia.

Follow-up brain scannings were normal except for the radioisotope accumulation apparently at the site of operation until February 1970 (Figure 61, center). Since the beginning of August 1970, however, dysphasia increased and a motor weakness developed on the right half of the body. Repeat brain scanning on August 25 showed a large, round and dense uptake with discrete margin in the left frontobasal region (Fig. 61, right). Angiography now disclosed tumor vessels with arteriovenous fistulas in the same region, associated with the appropriate dislocations of the vessels. Recraniotomy and left frontal lobectomy was performed for decompression, and this time histologic diagnosis was glioblastoma multiforme. The patient expired in March 1971, six months after the second operation.

In this patient, an initially positive scan turned out to be negative after operation and irradiation, thereafter, it changed again positive. The demonstration of positive uptake on the final scintigram evidently indicated the recurrence of tumor, both from the time course of serial studies and from the three dimensional shape and location of the radioactive focus.

The case of a teratocarcinoma in the right frontal lobe is illustrated in Figure 62. The patient, a 27-year-old man, was admitted in March 1970 on an emergency basis in semicomatose condition. He had had moderate fever and nuchal pain for two weeks, then developed right hemiparesis and decreased level of consciousness since several days prior to admission. Neurologic examination on admission disclosed left hemiparesis, bilateral choked discs, and marked nuchal rigidity. Right carotid angiography revealed a huge mass situated deeply in the right frontal lobe. A portion of the mass extended beneath the falx to the left of the midline.

Right frontal craniotomy was carried out immediately following angiography, and an encapsulated tumor measuring $4 \times 6 \times 6$ cm was totally removed. Histologic diagnosis was a teratocarcinoma.

After operation the patient showed a minimum hemiparesis on the left side, but papilledema subsided rapidly. Brain scanning first showed the superficial uptake in

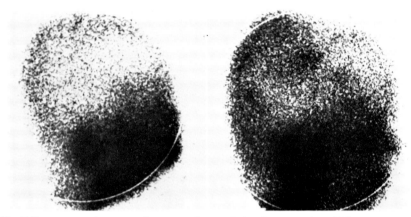

Fig. 62 Follow-up scans in a case of teratocarcinoma. *Left:* after operation; *Right:* recurrent tumor.

the right frontal area apparently due to the operative wound. Follow-up scans, however, restored rapidly to normal (Figure 62, left). Postoperative angiogram demonstrated the negative shift of the pericallosal artery.

In December 1970, the patient developed paralysis of upward gaze and became progressively somnolent. Repeat brain scanning now disclosed blurred but unequivocal abnormal uptake in the deep basofrontal and deep parietal regions (Figure 62, right). Angiography at that time again showed a negative shift of the internal cerebral vein, but in the lateral view, there was noted a downward displacement of the internal cerebral vein and deformation of the great vein of Galen. Positive contrast ventriculography revealed the filling defects in the trigone and the middle portion of the right lateral ventricle as well as the posterior third ventricle, confirming the presence of multiple tumors, probably due to dissemination along the cerebrospinal fluid pathways.

In this case, preoperative scanning could not be obtained so that the negative scan after operation did not necessarily rule out the presence of recurrent tumor. However, the final scintigram in December was clearly positive and the recurrence became evident. It should be stressed that the angiogram still demonstrated a negative shift of the pericallosal artery at that time.

Several points should be pointed out here for interpretation of the postoperative follow-up scans. Firstly, the operative wounds of scalp, skull and the brain cause the increased uptake of radioisotope for several months after operation. The radioactivity in the skull and scalp is superficial, and it is usually easy to differentiate from the more deeply seated tumor radioactivity. When the original lesion is located superficially, however, difficulty may be met and serial observations become necessary for differentiation between the two.

Secondly, if the tumor did not present the positive uptake before operation, its recurrence may not show the radioactive focus postoperatively. Similarly when the scanning was not performed before the operation, the interpretation of follow-up scan is rendered difficult, since the negative scan does not rule out the presence of the tumor.

Therefore, it is our policy to have the preoperative scan on hand for comparison and then perform the serial observations after operation with intervals. Single postoperative scan does not help so much and the importance of serial observations can not be over-emphasized.

Chapter IX

PEDIATRIC DISEASES

1. Congenital Hydrocephalus and Other Congenital Malformations

In the brain scanning of infants and children with congenital hydrocephalus, cranial vault which is seen as the peripheral band of radioactivity is disproportionately large compared to the facial structures (Figures 63 and 64). The area corresponding to the cerebral hemispheres is enlarged and shows exceptionally low background activity, apparently due to dilatation of the lateral ventricles. Low position of the transverse sinus and the torcular Herophili, and occasionally an asymmetry of the skull or abnormal configuration of the superior sagittal sinus may be noted by scanning. Thus, the brain scanning in the congenital hydrocephalus can indicate the enlargement of the supratentorial compartment but otherwise shows no distinctive findings.

Hydrocephalus in infancy and childhood may be secondary to the intracranial tumors. The choroid plexus papilloma is known to accompany the communicating type of hydrocephalus with few exceptions. Because of the extremely large size of the ventricles, pneumoencephalography or even ventriculography may fail to demonstrate the papilloma, especially when the bubble study is performed [136]. Since the choroid plexus takes up ^{99m}Tc pertechnetate, brain scanning with this agent is expected to reveal the choroid plexus papillomas with high accuracy.

In infancy and childhood, a significant number of intracerebral or extracerebral neoplasms other than the choroid plexus papillomas are also associated with hydrocephalus, which is usually obstructive in nature. Brain scanning in these cases may prove to be very useful in detecting the organic cause of the hydrocephalus. Figure 63

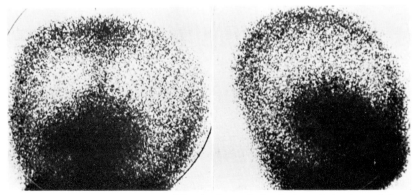

Fig. 63 Suprasellar teratoma resulting in the occlusive hydrocephalus in an infant. *Left:* frontal view; *Right:* right lateral view.

shows a brain scan of an infant in whom the bubble study failed to reveal the tumor and the ventriculoatrial shunt was performed previously. Months later, the head circumference showed a steady increase despite a well-functioning shunting device, and the brain scanning revealed a huge uptake at the base of the skull. At operation, a large teratoma was removed.

In Dandy-Walker syndrome the head is progressively enlarged with or without hydrocephalus. The torcular Herophili and the transverse sinuses are elevated and the transverse sinuses show a steep descent [166], which can be demonstrated by angiography, sinusography or by brain scanning [151, 166].

Hemicranial cysts or a large porencephalic cyst may show displacement of the superior sagittal sinus away from the involved hemisphere. The side of involvement has decreased radioactivity compared to the opposite side. These changes may be noted in frontal or occipital views of scintigrams but most prominently in vertex view.

Another important lesion which produces enlargement of the skull in children is the subdural effusion in which the ventricular enlargement is commonly found. Although the subdural effusion is usually easy to differentiate from congenital hydrocephalus by a simple procedure of subdural tap, brain scanning also may show the increased radioactivity in the peripheral rim in the frontal or occipital view (Figure 64).

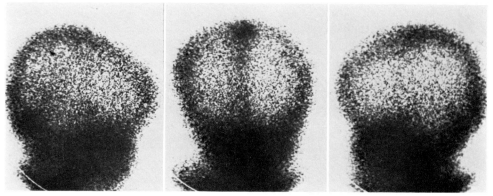

Fig. 64 Hydrocephalus associated with sundural effusion in an infant. *Left:* right lateral view; *Center:* frontal view; *Right,* left lateral view.

Mealey described in 1962 that the size and location of infantile subdural effusion could be accurately visualized by radioactive scanning after injection of the radionuclide directly into the subdural cavity [97]. For this procedure, small amounts of ^{131}I RISA, ^{99m}Tc pertechnetate or more recently [169]Yb DTPA are injected percutaneously into the subdural space. The radionuclide becomes distributed uniformly throughout the fluid collection, and can be localized by external detection (Figure 65).

The radiation dose with the subdural scanning has been measured and is within the acceptable levels. When 30 μCi of ^{131}I RISA are injected into the subdural space of an infant weighing 7 kg, a total body dose is 0.334 rad [100]. Moreover, the most of the injected radionuclide can be recovered by aspiration of the fluids as soon as scanning is completed, so that the local and whole body irradiation hazards are practically negligible.

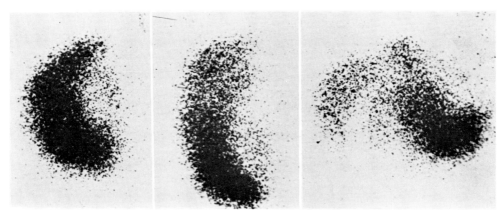

Fig. 65 Infantile subdural effusion over the right cerebral hemisphere. Subdural scintigrams with
[131]I RISA. *Left:* frontal view; *Center,* vertex view; *Right:* right lateral view.

The infantile subdural effusion may be unilateral, bilateral but independent, or bilateral and communicating. It may locate in the atypical area such as in the interhemispheric fissure and may show variable configurations. The angiogram can not adequately delineate the extent of the fluid collection, and the subdural air study may also fail to demonstrate the dimension of the effusion. The subdural scanning, on the other hand, has been found to be a safe and efficient technic in delineating the extent of the effusion, and is very useful as a guide in planning and following up the neurosurgical treatment of the patient.

Brain scanning in the meningocele and meningomyelocele usually does not help diagnosis. One exceptional case is shown in Figures 66 through 68. In this particular case the initial diagnosis was a meningomyelocele. Brain scanning, however, disclosed a dense uptake of radioisotope in the protruding mass in the cervicodorsal junction and at operation a solid mass was totally removed. Histologic diagnosis was a cavernous angioma.

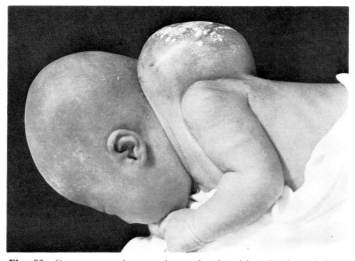

Fig. 66 Cavernous angioma at the cervico-dorsal junction in an infant.

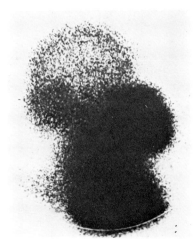

Fig. 67 Cavernous angioma at the cervicodorsal junction in an infant.
Lateral view of the head and chest.

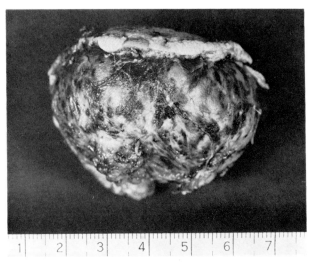

Fig. 68 Cavernous angioma at the cervico-dorsal junction in an infant.
Operative specimen.

2. Pediatric Brain Tumors

Brain tumors in pediatric age differ significantly from those in adults both in their histologic types and in their anatomical distribution. In adult, about 75 per cent of brain tumors are supratentorial, whereas in children, 60 per cent or more arise in the posterior cranial fossa [90].

Meningioma, metastatic carcinoma, pituitary adenoma, acoustic neurinoma and glioblastoma multiforme involving the cerebral hemisphere are common lesions in the adult, but they are extremely rare in children. On the other hand, the incidence of craniopharyngioma, pontine glioma, cerebellar astrocytoma and medulloblastoma is much higher in children (Table 7).

Over-all detection rate in pediatric brain tumors ranges from 50 to 70 per cent in

Table 7 Intracranial tumors in children (Matson[90])

Type of tumors	Number of cases
Astrocytoma grade I–II	202
Medulloblastoma	139
Brain stem glioma*	79
Craniopharyngioma	68
Ependymoma	66
Astrocytoma grade III–IV	64
Optic glioma	27
Choroid plexus papilloma	23
Dermoid cyst	12
Teratoma	11
Others	63
Total	754

*Many unverified.

the reported series [27, 98, 148], which is lower than expected in the adult series. The difference certainly is due partly to the size and location of the tumor, but it seems more dependent on the histologic character of the lesion [102].

3. Glioma of Brain Stem

One of the most common locations of gliomas in childhood is within the brain stem, namely the portion of the brain between the hypothalamus and the upper cervical cord. It accounts for 10.5 per cent (79 cases out of 750) of all intracranial tumors in the pediatric age, or about 19 per cent of infratentorial tumors in Matson's series (Table 8) [90]. Because of its unfavorable location, operation is rarely performed and the histologic diagnosis remains unknown in a large number of cases.

Table 8 Posterior fossa tumors in children (Matson[90])

Type of tumors	Number of cases
Cerebellar astrocytoma	134
Medulloblastoma	126
Brain stem glioma	78
Ependymoma	34
Mixed glioma of cerebellum	24
Dermoid cyst	10
Others	12
Total	418

Brain scans in the gliomas of brain stem are almost invariably negative and this poor result is practically the most important factor for the low detection rate of isotopic scanning method in the posterior fossa tumors in children. McAfee and Fueger [93] failed to localize the lesion in each of their six cases with ^{131}I RISA or ^{203}Hg chlormerodrin, Mishkin and Mealey [102] failed in all of their seven cases, Lincke [84] could obtain the abnormal scan in none of his five cases, and we have also experienced positive result in none of seven cases.

Although several authors have reported positive scans in a few cases of brain stem glioma [16, 44, 126, 148], the above-mentioned poor results in this lesion seem to suggest that, when an unequivocal positive scan is obtained, one should rather suspect a lesion other than the brain stem glioma. This is particularly important in the clinical practice, since the brain stem glioma is inoperable and always rapidly fatal, whereas other kinds of curable lesions may simulate this both clinically and radiologically.

Lincke [84] reported such an example in a four-year-old boy whose diagnosis on the first and second admissions was a pontine glioma. However, brain scanning in this boy revealed a dense accumulation of radioisotope in the median to left paramedian region of the posterior cranial fossa, and angiography later disclosed a meningioma.

4. Cerebellar Astrocytoma

Cerebellar astrocytoma is one of the most common tumors in childhood, accounting for 16 per cent in Gerlach's series [39], or 134 of 418 posterior fossa tumors in children in Matson's series (32 per cent) [90]. The tumor involves either cerebellar hemisphere or vermis, and often reaches an enormous size, but it is histologically well-differentiated and its progression is very slow and prognosis after surgery is invariably quite favorable. Indeed, this is the only glioma which can be cured by total removal. The tumor is often cystic with a mural nodule, but it may be totally solid.

Fortunately the accuracy of brain scanning in this benign tumor is quite excellent, and the detection rate reaches or well exceeds 90 per cent level in most reports [148].

The lesion is best seen in the occipital or angled posterior view as a dense and homogeneous radioactive focus below the torcular activity, and in the midline or laterally in the cerebellar hemisphere. In the lateral view, the lesion is seen below the radioactivity of torcular Herophili and in the posterior half of the posterior cranial fossa. Cystic or solid nature of the tumor does not seem to affect the pattern or intensity of the radioisotope accumulation (Figures 69 and 70).

5. Medulloblastoma

Medulloblastoma is a group of gliomas characteristically found in the posterior cranial fossa of children, arising usually in the region of the anterior medullary velum and occupying the midline cerebellar position. This tumor accounts for 18.0 per cent in

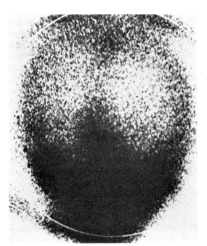

Fig. 69   Midline cerebellar astrocytoma. Occipital view.

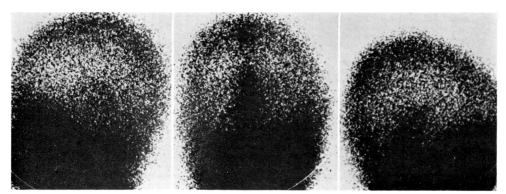

Fig. 70 Cerebellar astrocytoma extended through the tentorial notch into the supratentorial region. *Left:* left lateral view; *Center:* angled posterior view; *Right:* right lateral view.

Gerlach's series [39], and 18.5 per cent in Matson's series [90] of all intracranial tumors in the pediatric age, or 30 per cent of infratentorial tumors in his series.

Medulloblastoma usually reaches a considerable size before it becomes clinically manifest, and they are highly vascular and histologically undifferentiated. Nevertheless, they usually do not take up enough radionuclide to be detected by external scanning, and the detection rate in the reported series does not reach the 50 per cent level. Unfortunately we have experienced only 2 cases of medulloblastoma in the past three years, and the scanning was negative in one but it was positive in the other (Figure 71). Since medulloblastoma is so common in the pediatric age, its low detection rate is another reason for the low over-all diagnostic accuracy of the scanning technic in the posterior fossa tumors in childhood.

6. Ependymoma, Ependymoblastoma and Other Tumors

Ependymoma or ependymoblastoma of the fourth ventricle is an another important posterior fossa tumor in children. The majority of the cases can be localized by brain scanning, and when it is visualized its scan image, mainly in the midline cerebellum, is nonspecific and the differentiation from the medulloblastoma is impossible on the basis of scanning alone (Figures 72 and 73).

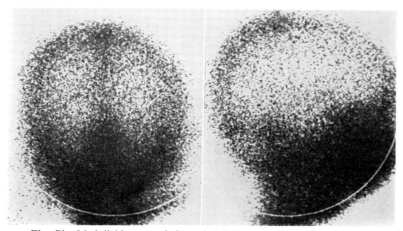

Fig. 71 Medulloblastoma. *Left:* occipital view; *Right:* right lateral view.

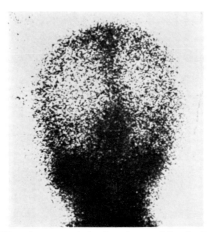

Fig. 72 Ependymoma of the fourth ventricle. Occipital view.

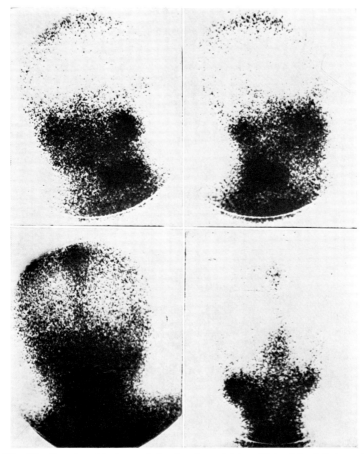

Fig. 73 Ependymoblastoma of the fourth ventricle. *Upper left:* left lateral view; *Upper right:* right lateral view; *Lower left:* Frontal view; and *Lower right:* Occipital view.

Mixed glioma of the cerebellum, dermoid and epidermoid tumors, sarcoma and choroid plexus papilloma, may be seen in the posterior cranial fossa of children. Incidence of these tumors is low and the experience of brain scanning is limited so that the diagnostic value of the scanning technic is not clear.

From the experience of brain scanning in the infratentorial tumors in children, it is evident that the scanning technic cannot be used as the sole diagnostic procedure. Scanning should always be considered an integral part of the neuroradiologic examinations in the pediatric patient suspected of harboring a mass lesion in the posterior fossa, and the result should be supplemented by additional methods of investigation.

Chapter X

OVER-ALL RESULTS OF BRAIN SCANNING IN INTRACRANIAL TUMORS

The over-all results in consecutive 152 cases encountered in the initial one year period are listed in Tables 9 and 11. The results are classified as positive or negative and the inconclusive cases are grouped with the negatives. In this period, most of the hospitalized patients were scanned for screening purposes, recently however, we have performed brain scanning intentionally selecting the patients suspected of harboring the mass lesion at the base of the brain or deep in the midline structures, so that the recent population does not seem to represent the average distribution of various kinds of pathologies.

Distribution of the results as a function of nature of the lesion is given in Table 9. It becomes evident from the table that 80 per cent of intracranial tumors showed a definite radioactive focus in the brain scan. Table clearly shows that the brain scanning demonstrates glioblastomas, meningiomas, and metastatic carcinomas most accurately, the over-all detection rate in these three histologic types of tumors being 93 per cent. On the other hand, the results are rather poor in gliomas of low grade malignancy, pituitary adenoma, craniopharyngioma or acoustic neurinoma. These results are generally in consonant with those of others, irrespective of radionuclides and instruments used (Table 10) [16, 30, 36, 92, 114, 143].

Distribution of positive results is correlated with the sites of the lesion in Table 11.

Table 9 Over-all results in 152 consecutive cases of proven brain tumors as related to the histology

Type of neoplasm	Number of cases	Brain scanning	
		Positive	Negative
Meningioma	26	24	2
Glioblastoma	21	19	2
Carcinoma	22	21	1
Astrocytoma and oligodendroglioma	23	18	5
Ependymoma	8	7	1
Neurinoma	8	5	3
Pituitary adenoma and craniopharyngioma	16	6	10
Deep, midline tumor	9	6	3
Miscellaneous	19	14	5
Total	152	120 (79.6%)	32

Table 10 Over-all results of scanning in the representative series by several authors

Authors	Year	Nuclide	Number of cases	Per cent correct
Sweet and Brownell[143]	1955	[74]As	131	76%
DiChiro[30]	1961	[131]I RISA	106	84
McAfee and Fueger[93]	1964	"	141	72
Bucy and Ciric[15,16]	1965	[203]Hg and [197]Hg Chlormerodrin	80	74
Overton et al.[114]	1965	"	100	80
Quinn et al.[119]	1965	[99m]Tc Per-technetate	66	83
Filson et al.[36]	1965	"	97	90
Handa et al.[53]	1969	"	152	80
Rasmussen et al.[124]	1970	"	501	70

Table 11 Over-all scan results in 152 consecutive cases of proven brain tumors as related to the location

Site of lesion	Number of cases	Brain scanning	
		Positive	Negative
Supratentorial (Excluding basal region)	103	92	11
Sellar region	33	18	15
Infratentorial	12	7	5
Multiple	4	3	1
Total	152	120	32

Locations of the tumor are arbitrarily classified into four groups:

1) the supratentorial tumors excluding those in the basal location,

2) supratentorial tumors near or at the base of the brain such as craniopharyngioma, pituitary adenoma or chordoma,

3) posterior fossa tumors and

4) multiple tumors.

The table clearly demonstrates the well-known difficulty encountered in detecting the tumors in the basal, sellar and suprasellar location as well as the infratentorial tumors.

The poor results in the basal or infratentorial tumors seem to be due to several factors. First of all, the size of the lesion tends to be smaller when compared to the hemispheric mass. The tumor locating in the basal or infratentorial region shows cranial nerve signs or increase in the intracranial pressure early in their growth and comes to the study while the size of the mass is still rather small, while the supratentorial, hemipheric tumor tends to be larger when it becomes symptomatic.

Secondly, the high background radioactivity of the temporal and occipital muscles makes the detection of basal tumors difficult. The undesirable effect of background activity is clearly shown by the fact that all of five cases with negative scans among 69 glioblastomas, meningiomas and metastatic carcinomas were in the temporal lobe or at the base of the middle fossa.

Thirdly, the radioisotopic accumulation is poor and the focus-to-brain uptake ratio might be actually low in the basal tumors, as is often the case in craniopharyngiomas or epidermoids.

Over-all accuracy in a series of patients thus varies considerably depending on the distribution of types and locations of tumors in the materials. In our experience during the first one year period, the detection rate was approximately 80 per cent, whereas recently the rate has decreased to less than 70 per cent. This is attributed to our intentional selection of the cases with tumors in the suprasellar, retrosellar or midline location for experimental trial of computer data display. It follows naturally that we should be careful in comparing the results of different authors, the composition of each series as a function of the type of the pathologies and of the locations of the lesions must be taken into serious consideration.

Moreover, there is no objective criteria whereby one can classify a given scintigram as positive, negative or equivocal. A certain number of scintigrams look pathologic in one view only and not in others. Some may categorize such a case as positive, some as negative or equivocal. The amounts of clinical and radiological informations inevitably affect the scan interpretation, particularly in the marginal cases. When one knows that the focal electroencephalographic abnormality exists in a given case, one tends to interpret otherwise normal or equivocal scintigram as pathologic. When the scintigrams are overread, the selectivity of brain scanning increases but the false negative scan also increases, and the result is a marked impairment of usefulness of brain scanning for the screening purposes.

Chapter XI

DIFFERENTIAL DIAGNOSIS

Although radioisotope scanning of the brain was originally considered a method of detection of brain tumors, it became apparent that abnormal uptake of radioisotope could be noted in a multitude of non-neoplastic lesions including the cerebral infarction, intracerebral hematoma, brain abscess, arteriovenous malformation, aneurysm, encephalitis, cerebritis and granulomas, acute phase of multiple sclerosis, leukemic infiltrates, vasculitis, cerebral contusion and edema, radiation necrosis and several other pathologic conditions. Extracerebral diseases such as scalp wound, metastatic deposits in the scalp and the skull, extracerebral hematoma, osteomyelitis, fibrous dysplasia, Paget's disease, and several other disease processes also can produce positive scans. It seems to be worthwhile at this point, therefore, to consider whether there exists any possibility of differentiating one kind of lesion from another on the basis of brain scanning.

In distinguishing the nature of the lesion in a given patient, there are number of valuable radioisotopic techniques which can be applied. These include section scanning, computer scanning, radionuclide angiography, radioisotopic transit and washout studies, macroaggregates perfusion scanning, and sequential or serial scanning. Some of them need the special instrumentation, programming and the trained personnel, but others can be performed as the routine procedure, and we feel that the planned sequential scanning carried out and interpreted by the experienced staff is of significant value in the differential diagnosis of a multitude of cerebral and extracerebral lesions.

For the purpose of the differential diagnosis, following factors should be considered:
1) size and shape of the abnormal uptake of radioisotope;
2) contour of margin of the radioactive focus;
3) density and homogeneity of the radioisotope accumulation;
4) number of, or multiplicity of the lesions;
5) location of the focus;
6) time course of positive uptake in the sequential scanning; and
7) temporal factors in serial studies performed with the intervals in between of a few days to weeks.

1. Size and Shape of Abnormal Uptake
The positive uptake may be round or spherical, ovoid, bandlike or linear, irregular, crescentic or wedge-shaped. The shape of the uptake should be studied at least in the two planes.

Classically, most tumors present a spherical or ovoid shape of radioisotope uptake, but they can be quite irregular in shape especially in gliomas of high maligmancy.

As a rule, intracerebral hematoma, granuloma, brain abscess also show more or less ovoid uptake.

The positive uptake in cerebral infarction has been described to be wedge-shaped on the lateral view and crescentic on the frontal or occipital view. This differs from the tumor in that the uptake of a cerebral infarct does not cross the midline. In the first two days after a stroke, brain edema can shift midline structures to the opposite side but the scan of the edematous brain is negative at this time.

However, the crescentic and wedge-shaped uptake is not the rule but rather infrequent, and the uptake is more frequently irregular and band-like or ovoid on the lateral view, and occasionally quite round and spherical.

2. *Density and Homogeneity of Focus*

Generalization is that the accumulation of the radioactivity tends to be quite dense and homogeneous in certain kinds of tumors, especially in meningiomas, metastases and glioblastomas, while it is less dense in brain abscesses, intracerebral hematomas, and a number of astrocytomas and other kinds of gliomas of low malignancy.

Cerebral infarctions usually present the focus with less density, but the scintigraphic quality of the focus varies widely according to the age of the lesion.

3. *Number of Lesions*

While there are exceptions, detection of multiple foci of radioisotope uptake must be taken always as a sign of metastatic lesions, particularly when the foci are found wide apart on both hemispheres, or, one in the supratentorial region and the other infratentorially.

Another multiple lesions which may be encountered are the multiple brain abscesses of cardiac origin. It is perfectly possible to find contusions or infarctions in the multiple sites. In gliomas, solitary metastasis or several other kinds of tumors, necrosis or hemorrhage of a part of tumor often appears cool, and the scintigram may show seemingly separated foci of radioactivity in the viable portions of the neoplasm.

Chronic subdural hematomas may be found bilaterally, and this constitutes, in a sense, another group of double foci. When bilateral, symmetrical crescent-like activities in the frontal or occipital view sometimes makes diagnosis difficult.

4. *Location of Focus*

Location of the focus in the scan is one of the most important criteria for differentiation of neoplastic and non-neoplastic lesions, and also between the kinds of tumors involving the brain. Ninety per cent of cerebral infarctions occur in the territory of the middle cerebral artery, either due to embolization or to thrombosis of the middle cerebral artery or of the internal carotid artery. The middle cerebral artery supplies most of the lateral convex surface of the cerebral hemisphere, and the infarction does not cross the line of boundary between this artery and the anterior or posterior cerebral artery.

Anterior cerebral infarctions are quite rare, when found the radioactivity is found in the frontal parasagittal area. Posterior cerebral infarction is found in the parieto-occipital region, where the tumors are relatively uncommon. Infarctions in the vertebrobasilar system do not present the positive scans with few exceptions.

If the radioactive focus does not conform to the area of territory of the one cerebral artery and exceeds the line of boundary, it is most likely to be a tumor. Since most infarctions are superficial lesions involving the cortical and subcortical tissues, the lesion which locates deeply in the brain and does not reach the surface area is likely to be a tumor than an infarction, but the exceptions are reported in the occlusion of the striate vessels or the artery of Heubner.

When the increased radioactivity extends onto the contralateral side across the midline, it is very likely to indicate a neoplasm, representing either the shift of the midline or the extension into the contralateral cerebral hemisphere. When the glioblastoma involves both hemispheres crossing the corpus callosum, angiographic determination of true extent of the tumor often proves difficult, but the frontal or occipital view of the brain scanning reveals a typical butterfly pattern of radioisotope uptake which is diagnostic in most cases. A falx meningioma could also produce a somewhat similar appearance but the radioactive focus tends to be round rather than butterfly-shaped, and more distinct in its margin. Parasagittal meningioma and meningioma arising from the cribriform plate often produce the foci on either side of the midline, but their typical locations greatly help the diagnosis.

Frontal parasagittal lesions or the midline lesions at the frontal pole or the base of the anterior cranial fossa are mostly neoplastic, infarctions being quite rare in these regions. In the subfrontal and suprasellar region, meningioma is the most probable diagnosis. Although the suprasellar extension of pituitary adenoma or the glioma of the optic nerve and hypothalamus may produce the positive uptake, they are usually less dense and less distinct in margin.

Infarctions in the vertebro-basilar system rarely cause radioisotope uptake so that the positive scan in the infratentorial region is indicative of neoplastic nature of the lesion. The foci which appear in both the middle and posterior cranial fossae are tumors, especially meningiomas arising from the tentorium or the petrous ridge.

Deeply situated focus which apparently corresponds to one of the ventricles, especially the lateral ventricle, would indicate the neoplasm. Both thalamic tumor and capsular hemorrhage present rather blurred uptake of radioisotope and their differentiation is difficult or practically impossible on the basis of brain scanning.

5. *Time Course of Uptake in Sequential Scanning*

In addition to the morphological characteristics such as the size, shape, margin, location, density, homogeneity and multiplicity of the radioactive foci, time course of positive uptake of radioisotope in the pathologic focus is of great value in differentiating the various kinds of disease processes on the basis of scan images. Such a dynamic study with sequential imaging of radioisotopic distribution has been made practical for the first time with introduction of the short-lived radionuclide and a gamma-ray scintillation camera.

Several authors studied the chronologic patterns of radioisotope uptake in various kinds of organic intracranial lesions and correlated them with the nature of the pathologies. Schlesinger and coworkers [139] in 1962 stated that the lesions which are rich in the blood content and flow such as arteriovenous malformations and angioblastic meningiomas were best shown on the scintigrams immediately after injection of ^{131}I RISA. Meningiomas in general presented the clear foci of radioactive tracers within 24 hours, whereas in most gliomas the positive uptake appeared somewhat later. Astrocytomas of low grade malignancy which were mostly poorly vascularized showed less intense radioactivity. In many cystic lesions, the accumulation of radioactivity was delayed to appear and the scintigrams of best qualities were obtained only at 48 hours postinjection or even later.

Similarly using ^{131}I RISA as a tracer but based on the numerical data, Planiol [116] classified pathologic foci into several groups. In order to describe the characteristics of the radioisotope uptake, she defined main variables as follows. The *"maximum intensity"* was defined as the highest reading in the focus, calculated against a corresponding point which, in most cases was the symmetrical point of the cerebral hemisphere on the contralateral side. Information as to the relative penetration speed of the tracer agent and also on the storage capacity in reference to time of the lesions for ^{131}I RISA were obtained from a survey of the intensity versus time after injection of ^{131}I RISA through the successive studies.

A focus observed during the first half hour following administration of the radioisotope and which did not increase in intensity during the next 24–48 hours was called *"immediate and stable"* focus. A focus which became very evident in 1 and 4 hours, and then increased moderately up to 24 hours after injection was called *"early"* and a focus which did not appear within three hours but became visible next day, or whose moderate initial intensity increased by more than 50 per cent in the interval of 24 hours was called *"delayed"* or *"late."*

The distribution of hyperactivity of the focus showed a variation of wide range. For practical purposes, to characterize a focus as *"clear,"* Planiol evaluated the ratio between the number of positions with a count rate equal to or greater than 40 per cent, and the total number of positions occupied by that focus, and in the case of less intense focus, with a maximum rate under 40 per cent, the ratio between the surface occupied by this maximum, if clearly marked, and the total surface of the focus. The focus was classified as *"well circumscribed"* or *"clear"* when the ratio was over 0.2 and as *"blurred"* or *"poorly defined"* when it was equal to or less than 0.2.

Combining these temporal and spatial factors in the distribution of ^{131}I RISA, Planiol studied the main characteristics in 100 cases in each of four kinds of neoplasms, namely glioblastoma, meningioma, astrocytoma and metastasis. In meningiomas, 76 of 100 cases presented the early and clear focus, and 13 showed clear but delayed, three blurred and early, and in eight clear and early focus.

Astrocytomas showed similar results; 62 belonged to delayed and blurred group, 22 blurred and early group, six clear and delayed and in 10 the focus appeared early and was cool.

In metastases, the foci were classified as clear in 87 cases, in 71 of them they were delayed and in 16 early. In 10 more cases, the foci were grouped as delayed and blurred, and in three early and blurred. The predominances observed were so striking that the phrases were introduced; *"a focus of the meningioma type"* for an early and clear focus, *"metastatic type"* for delayed and clear focus, or *"glioblastoma type"* for a delayed and blurred focus.

The early and clear focus actually corresponded to a meningioma in 74 per cent of cases, although in 20 per cent it was seen in the malignant tumors, either glioblastoma or metastasis. The delayed and blurred focus indicated glioblastoma in 72 per cent, whereas in 11 per cent it was seen in astrocytomas. In delayed and clear type of focus, the results were relatively poor. Although the most frequent pathologies were metastases (52 per cent), 26 were diagnosed as glioblastoma or astrocytoma. The early and blurred focus was the least frequent and was found mostly in gliomas (76 per cent).

In hematomas, a hyperactive area covered a large area of the hemicranium; it was blurred and was described as "*en plateau variety.*" Abscess characteristically showed a delayed appearance of rather clear focus.

From these results, Planiol concluded that the etiology of the radioactive focus could be foreseen with reasonable certainty on the basis of gamma-encephalographic analysis.

Results of serial brain scanning with ^{197}Hg or ^{203}Hg chlormerodrin were described by Economos and coworkers [35]. In meningiomas, they found the highest radioisotope uptake one to two hours after injection. Thereafter, the radioactivity in the hot foci decreased gradually. Gliomas were noted as the early active foci, but the radioisotope uptake increased with time and the lesion often remained clear for 24 hours or longer. Non-neoplastic lesions such as brain abscesses, cerebral infarctions and intracerebral hematomas, also demonstrated a progressive accumulation of the tracer, but the focal accumulation of radioactivity was much less than in gliomas.

Also using ^{197}Hg chlormerodrin and by automatic contour scanner, Yamamoto and Feindel [168] repeated examinations twice or three times within a period of 24 hours after injection of the radioactive nuclide and the changes in the differential uptake were determined. In glioblastomas, they found that the turnover rate in the tumor was much slower and less linear than that of the background radioactivity in the normal brain, and the differential uptake showed a rapid increase. In meningiomas, the uptake ratio reached a maximum within a short time and then became stable within three to six hours. In angiomas the turnover rates in the tumor and the brain tissue were similar, and the differential uptake decreased rapidly with time. In cerebral infarctions the results were less uniform; in some cases the turnover was slow as in glioblastoma but in others, it showed similar pattern as seen in meningioma. Differential uptake, however, showed a more or less acute rise with time.

The results of our studies of sequential scintiphotography using a gamma-ray scintillation camera and ^{99m}Tc pertechnetate generally compare favorably with these previous studies [52, 53, 57]. We intravenously injected ^{99m}Tc pertechnetate in dosis of 10 mCi in an average adult patient. Following the serial study of first circulation of the isotope bolus through the brain (radionuclide angiography), sequential scintiphotographs were obtained 0.5 to 1, 3, 5, 10, 30, 45, 60 minutes, and occasionally 90 and 120 minutes, after injection, without moving the head of the patient and accumulating 10×10^4 to 15×10^4 counts for each exposure. At the same time interval, accumulation of counts for 60 seconds each were performed using a 1,600 channel multiparameter analyzer, and the data were stored in the magnetic tape system.

From among the sequential scintiphotographs, the one in which the focus was best shown was chosen and the corresponding count rate data were replayed and rearranged in 40 by 40 matrices. Referring to the original scintiphotography and the count rate sheet, the uptake ratio was calculated as follows:

$$\text{Uptake ratio} = \frac{F}{B} \text{ (arbitrary unit),}$$

where F = total counts in the matrix of three by three which presented maximum count rates in the pathologic focus, B = total counts in the matrix of three by three which showed the minimum count rates in the apparently normal portion of the brain.

Uptake ratios were calculated for the rest of the sequential studies using the same co-ordinates for the two sets of three by three matrices, one for the lesion and the other for the normal brain.

The chronologic patterns of sequential scintiphotography are classified into three main types. The lesion of *Type 1* is characterized by the focus which shows best demarcated and dense accumulation of radioactivity in the earliest phase followed by a more or less rapid decrease. Arteriovenous malformation, racemose and cavernous angiomas and meningiomas presented the foci of this type.

In Figure 74, sequential scintigrams in a case of arteriovenous malformation in the

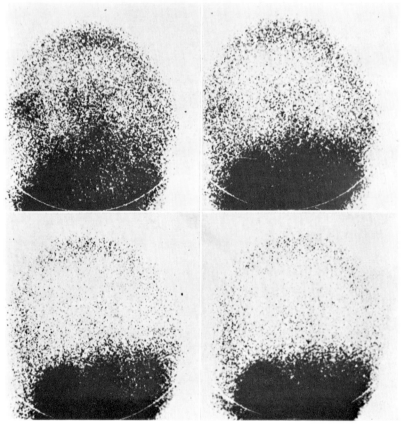

Fig. 74 Arteriovenous malformation in the sylvian region. *Upper left:* immediately after; *Upper right:* five minutes; *Lower left:* 30 minutes; and *Lower right:* 60 minutes after administration of ^{99m}Tc pertechnetate. Right lateral view.

sylvian region are illustrated. Immediately after intravenous injection of ^{99m}Tc per-technetate, an arteriovenous malformation and the torcular Herophili which on the preceding angiogram was seen to collect the blood from the malformation, were best seen. Five minutes later, however, radioactivity in both the arteriovenous anomaly and the torcular Herophili had decreased and the foci were much blurred in appearance. Thirty to 60 minutes after injection, the scintigrams were essentially normal, and no significant focal accumulation of radioactivity was noted in the brain. If the scintigrams were obtained only in the delayed phase following administration of the tracer, the lesion in this case might have escaped detection.

Other examples of sequential scintigrams in arteriovenous malformation are shown in Figures 75 and 76.

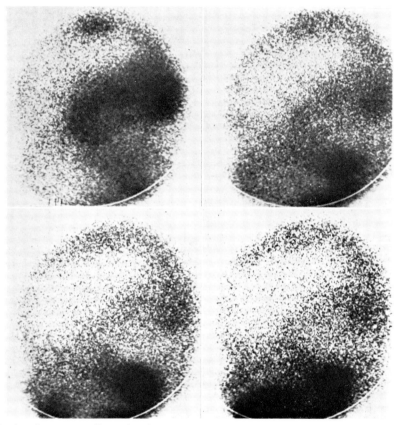

Fig. 75 Arteriovenous malformation in the left temporo-occipital region. *Upper left:* immediately after; *Upper right:* five minutes; *Lower left:* 15 minutes; and *Lower right:* 60 minutes after injection of ^{99m}Tc pertechnetate. Left lateral view.

Sequential scintigrams in a case of convexity meningioma in the right parieto-occipital region are shown in Figure 77. The focus was round, dense and best demarcated as typical of meningioma, again immediately after administration of ^{99m}Tc pertechnetate. Thereafter, the decrease in focal accumulation of radioactivity was very rapid and in scintigrams obtained 30–45 minutes after injection, it seemed difficult to predict the nature of the lesion.

Figure 78 illustrates sequential studies in another case of meningioma.

Arteriovenous anomalies always showed the maximum radioactivity in the earliest phase of sequential scintiphotographs. Thereafter, the abnormal concentration of radioactivity showed an acute decrease, and later scintiphotographs tended to normalize rapidly. Although serial angiography which provides precise anatomical information

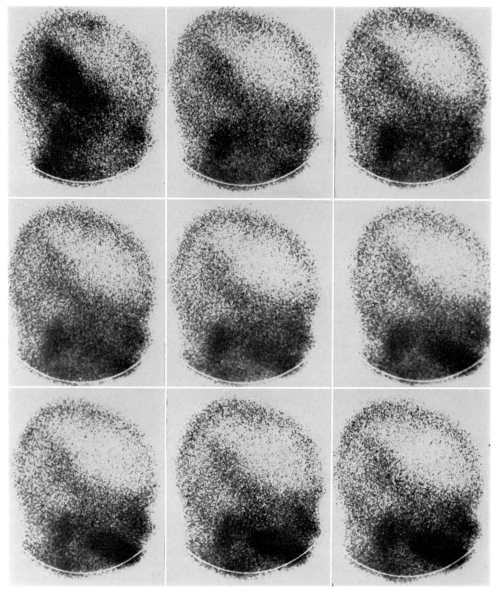

Fig. 76 Arteriovenous malformation. Sequential scintigrams from *Upper left:* immediately after injection of ^{99m}Tc pertechnetate to *Lower right:* 60 minutes later. Right lateral view.

of the lesion is indispensable for diagnosis and proper management of arteriovenous anomalies, all 21 cases of arteriovenous anomalies encountered in the present series showed definite scintigraphic abnormalities so far as being studied shortly after administration of the radionuclide.

In meningiomas, and also in a case of cavernous angioma of the brain, the chronologic pattern of sequential scintiphotography was essentially similar to that of arteriovenous anomalies. Although the focus in most cases remained hot during the period of sequential imaging for up to 120 minutes after injection, a fall in radioactivity was

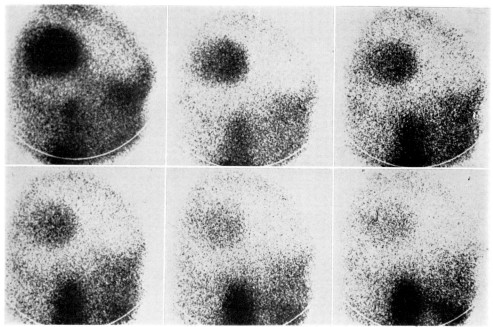

Fig. 77 Convexity meningioma. *Upper left:* immediately after; *Upper center:* five minutes; *Upper right:* 10 minutes; *Lower left:* 15 minutes; *Lower center:* 30 minutes; and *Lerwer right:* 45 minutes after injection. Right lateral view.

so rapid in some cases that the scintigrams tended to become essentially negative at the end of the study.

Glioma of low grade malignancy, cerebral infarctions and brain abscesses generally showed a pattern of progressive accumulation of radioactivity and were grouped as *Type 2* lesions.

Figure 79 illustrates a typical pattern in a case of astrocytoma involving the insular portion of the brain. The scintigram was equivocal immediately after administration of ^{99m}Tc pertechnetate, fifteen minutes after administration, a blurred radioisotope uptake was noted in the central region. After this, the uptake increased gradually and later showed an increasingly clear focus.

In the acute phase of cerebral infarction illustrated in Figure 80, carotid angiography demonstrated an avascular area surrounded by a perifocal capillary blush in the right parieto-occipital region. The scintigram taken shortly after administration of ^{99m}Tc pertechnetate revealed a cold central focus. The radioactivity in this central area increased gradually and reached a maximum degree at the end of the sequential studies up to 120 minutes after injection. Meanwhile the peripheral zone decreased in its initial increased radioactivity so that the *"doughnut"* appearance as seen in the initial phase was lost.

Gliomas and sarcomas generally showed the active focus in the early phase, but the radioactivity tended to further increase with time. Figure 81 shows an example. In metastatic carcinomas, the chronologic pattern of radioisotope uptake is less uniform. The uptake showed a progressive increase in the majority of cases (Figure 82), but the regressive course was noted in some instances (Figures 83 and 84).

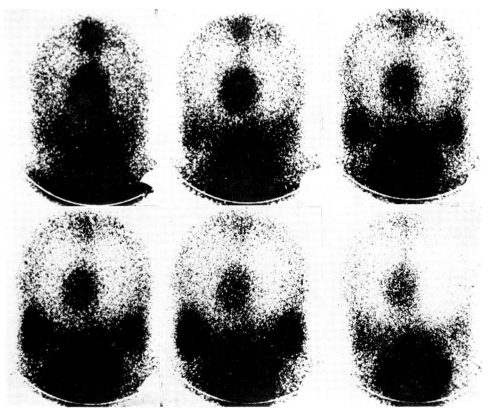

Fig. 78   Parasagittal meningioma. Frontal view. *Upper left:* immediately after; *Upper center:* five minutes; *Upper right:* 15 minutes; *Lower left:* 30 minutes; *Lower center:* 60 minutes; and *Upper right:* 90 minutes after injection.

As far as the sequential scintiphotographs are concerned, gliomas in general showed a progressive accumulation of radioactivity up to two hours after administration of the tracer.   However, there were noted several cases of gliomas in which the highest accumulation of radioactivity was demonstrated immediately after injection, which was followed by a rapid regression.   In one case the lesion proved to be glioblastoma, but in two, diagnosis was oligodendroglioma and no malignancy was seen histologically (Figure 85).   One common factor for each of these atypical cases was an intense tumor stain with obvious arteriovenous shunts as revealed by angiography.

Type 3 lesions comprise those lesions in which the focus remains persistently cold during the course of sequential studies.   This has been encountered in large cystic mass or intracerebral hematoma.   Occasionally, areas of central necrosis or hemorrhage into the tumor may appear cool but in most cases they tend to become hot with time and the persistently cold foci are extremely rare.

When the uptake ratios are determined numerically, their chronologic patterns are grouped into four, as shown in Figure 86.

Group 1 corresponds to *Type 1* lesion on sequential scintiphotographs and includes arteriovenous anomalies, angioma and meningioma.   In arteriovenous anomalies, the uptake ratio showed the maximum value in the initial read-out (0.5–1.5 minutes post-injection) following administration of ^{99m}Tc pertechnetate.   Thereafter, the ratio de-

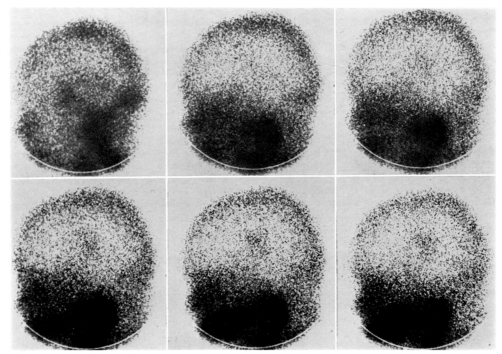

Fig. 79 Astrocytoma. Sequential scintigrams *Upper left:* immediately after; *Upper center:* five minutes; *Upper right:* 15 minutes; *Lower left:* 30 minutes; *Lower center:* 60 minutes; and *Lower right:* 120 minutes after injection. Left lateral view.

creased rapidly and reached the plateau in 10–15 minutes. The absolute values of maximum uptake ratio were scattered widely and this seemed to be due to differences in the size of the blood pool in the pathologic foci.

In most meningiomas and angioma, the uptake ratio showed an initial increase for several minutes, reached the maximum value in five to 10 minutes, then decreased more or less steeply. Exceptionally in a single case of meningioma the uptake curve was similar to that expected in arteriovenous malformation. Another one case was quite unusual and the uptake ratio showed a progressive increase for more than 60 minutes.

In *Group 4*, the uptake ratio remained below a unit. This group corresponds to the *Type 3* focus in sequential scintiphotography.

Type 2 foci are subdivided into two groups. *Group 2* comprises benign gliomas, cerebral infarctions and brain abscesses. The uptake ratio increased linearly throughout the course of the study or increased for 30–60 minutes and reached the plateau, but it never decreased during the period of study for two hours. In two cases of highly vascular oligodendroglioma stated before, the uptake curve exceptionally showed a regressive curve much the same as seen in arteriovenous malformation.

In *Group 3*, the uptake ratio showed an initial increase for 30–60 minutes which was followed by a secondary decrease. Most glioblastomas, metastatic carcinomas and sarcomas presented this pattern. Again, in one case of intracranial extension of carcinoma of the ethmoid sinus, the uptake ratio showed a regressive pattern as seen in meningioma. In this particular case, the preceding angiogram showed an enormous

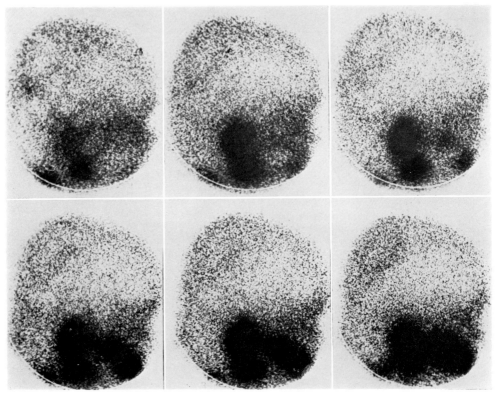

Fig. 80 Cerebral infarction. Right lateral view. *Upper left:* immediately after; *Upper center:* 15 minutes; *Upper right:* 30 minutes; *Lower left:* 45 minutes; *Lower center:* 60 minutes; and *Lower right:* 120 minutes after injection.

tumor vascularity supplied from the ophthalmic artery. The tumor stain persisted throughout the venous phase of angiography and the angiographical diagnosis was frontobasal meningioma.

Thus, our results of sequential scintiphotography and determination of the uptake ratio generally compare favorably with the previous studies mentioned above. In summary, the regressive course of radioisotope uptake was seen most often in arteriovenous anomalies, meningiomas and angioma. A few cases of glioma and metastatic carcinoma also showed the similar pattern. When the uptake ratios were determined by use of a 1,600 channel analyzer, chronologic patterns of differential uptake were somewhat different between the arteriovenous anomalies and meningiomas. In arteriovenous anomalies, the uptake ratio showed the highest value immediately after intravenous administration of ^{99m}Tc pertechnetate, whereas in most cases of meningiomas, the uptake ratio increased for five to 10 minutes before it reached the maximum level.

In no cases of arteriovenous anomalies in the present series, were there noted recent hemorrhages. Meningiomas demonstrated typical tumor stain on the angiogram, and in the exceptional cases of glioma or carcinoma which showed a regressive course of radioisotope uptake, carotid angiography demonstrated tumors with extremely high vascularity associated with early filling of the draining veins. In all of these cases, a large amount of ^{131}I MAA injected into the carotid artery was entrapped in the tumor and the pulmonary scanning often revealed the presence of arteriovenous

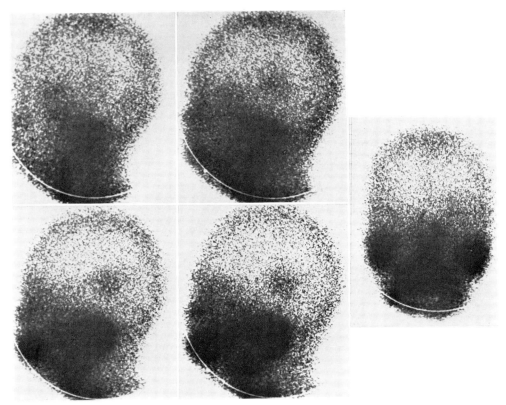

Fig. 81 Glioblastoma multiforme. *Upper left:* immediately after; *Upper right:* five minutes; *Lower left:* 45 minutes; and *Lower right:* 60 minutes after injection. Left lateral view. *Right:* Frontal view.

shunts (Figure 87). In ^{133}Xe scanning and flow determinations, rapid clearance in the focus also indicated the increased blood flow with or without associated arteriovenous short-circuit in the tumor.

Several factors have been considered to contribute to the differential accumulation of substances in the pathologic cerebral focus, including the increased vascularity and blood content, structural abnormalities of the neoplastic blood vessels, changes in the selective permeability between the blood and the brain, cellular or intercellular concent- ration of substances, metabolic demands of neoplastic cells, pinocytosis, osmolarity of fluid contents of hematoma or cysts, and others. Among them, a regressive course of radioisotope uptake seems to be dependent on the increased vascularity and blood content of the focus and not necessarily on the histologic nature of the lesion itself. In the highly vascular lesions with numerous distended blood vessels, a large quantity of radioactive tracers accumulate in the lesion at a time when the concentration in the blood is high, immediately after injection of the radionuclide. The brain scan be- comes positive and the differential uptake high, and this early visualization of the focus is caused by tracer-laden blood which is pooled in the vascular bed in the lesion.

In cases where the large blood pool is the main, if not exclusive, factor in the ac- cumulation of the radioactivity, then the chronologic course of the differential uptake should follow an ever decreasing pattern as seen in pure vascular malformations [18].

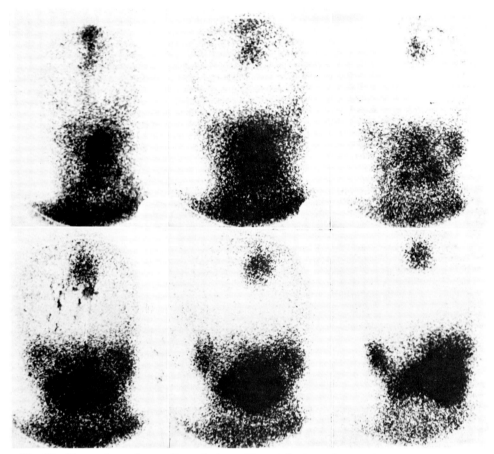

Fig. 82   Metastatic carcinoma. Frontal view. *Upper left:* immediately after; *Upper center:* five
minutes; *Upper right:* 30 minutes; *Lower left:* 60 minutes; *Lower center:* 90 minutes; and
Lower right: 120 minutes after injection of ^{99m}Tc pertechnetate.

In most meningiomas and other highly vascular tumors, however, there seems to
exist an additional mechanism of radioisotope uptake, which modifies the uptake curve
in various degrees.

In *Group 4* lesions, ^{133}Xe clearance studies and ^{131}I MAA perfusion scanning showed
clearly that the focus was poor in blood flow and vascular bed.   Angiography revealed
an avascular mass, and radionuclide angiography also disclosed the area of poor perfusion.   All these data suggest that the focus is poor in blood content, which is represented in a persistently low (less than a unit) uptake of radioactivity in the
sequential studies.

In *Group 2* foci with a progressive increase in radioisotope uptake, increased vascularity
does not seem to play any significant role.   In no case carotid angiography showed the
tumor vascularity. ^{133}Xe and ^{131}I MAA studies also proved the poor perfusion in the
focus.   In this group of pathologies, therefore, changes in the selective permeability in
the tumor and perifocal edematous brain seem to be the main causative factors in
the progressive accumulation of ^{99m}Tc pertechnetate on sequential scintiphotographs.

Group 3 lesions were more variable.   In most cases, however, ^{133}Xe clearance studies

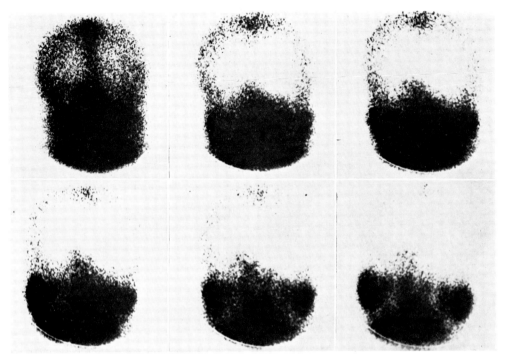

Fig. 83: Carcinoma arose from the frontal sinus. Frontal view. *Upper left:* immediately after; *Upper center:* 15 minutes; *Upper right:* 30 minutes; *Lower left:* 45 minutes; *Lower center:* 60 minutes; and *Lower right:* 120 minutes after injection.

and ^{131}I MAA perfusion scanning showed an increase in tumor blood flow, which was supported by angiographic features as well as operative findings. It seems, therefore, that both the increased blood content in the tumor and the local loss or breakdown of the barrier mechanism contribute to the chronologic pattern of an initial increase followed by a secondary decrease as seen in isotope uptake curves. It seems interesting to note that the lesions of this group were malignant tumors, known to contain abnormal neoplastic vessels; thin-walled arteries with poorly defined muscular layer, tortuous, lacunar and aneurysmal dilatations, glomeruloid formations and arteriovenous shunts [47, 108, 138, 167].

It is concluded, therefore, that the vascularity and blood content of the focus are the important factors in determining the chronologic course of isotope uptake in the brain scanning with ^{99m}Tc pertechnetate. Of course, morphologic factors, density and homogeneity of the isotope accumulation, multiplicity and the location of the lesion provide useful informations as to the nature of the lesions. In addition, dynamic study of focal isotope uptake by means of sequential scintiphotography not only increases the rate of positive scanning but also substantially aids in the specific diagnosis of nature of the pathologic foci.

6. Temporal Factors

Time relationship between the onset of clinical symptoms and the time of scanning adds important information about the pathologic nature of the lesion. Especially it is of great value in the differentiation of neoplastic and non-neoplastic disease processes.

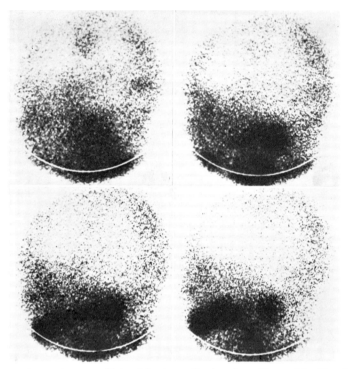

Fig. 84 Metastatic carcinoma. *Upper left:* immediately after; *Upper right* 20 minutes; *Lower left:* 60 minutes; and *Lower right:* 120 minutes after injection. Left lateral view.

In general, the neoplastic focus which once showed the positive uptake of radioisotope does not tend to become negative on the repeat scanning carried out days to weeks later using the same tracer agent. The radioactive focus either increases both in the size and the intensity of accumulation, or it remains the same. A rare exception is the case associated with the hemorrhage into the tumor, in which the initial large focus of radioisotope uptake may reduce in size, with the resolution of the hematoma, but the repeat scan does not usually restore to normal.

Cerebral infarction, on the other hand, may present a negative scan for the initial several days to a week, after that the rate of positive scan increases so that the 70–80 per cent of infarctions show the positive uptake during the second to fourth week after the onset of the clinical symptoms. Thereafter, the positivity again decreases and it is rare to obtain the positive scan at the sixth week or later.

Accordingly, when the initial positive scan restores to normal in the repeat studies in the course of a few weeks, the causative lesion is most probably cerebral infarction rather than the neoplastic lesion. Since the differentiation between the cerebral infarction and the brain tumor is not necessarily possible on the basis of morphologic characteristics of the focus alone, the serial scanning is an essential part of the scintigraphic study in clarifying the disease etiology. It should be stressed here, however, that rarely a positive scan due to a massive cerebral infarction may persist several months to even a year after the onset. Another important fact is that the occurrence of positive scan in the patient with a cerebrovascular lesion by no means excludes the presence of the neoplasm.

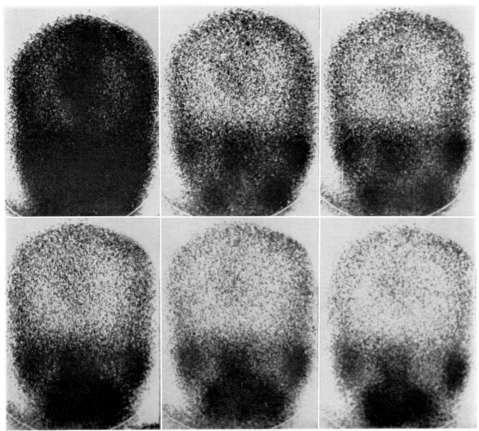

Fig. 85 Highly vascular oligodendroglioma. *Upper left:* immediately after; *Upper center:* 15 minutes after; *Upper right:* 30 minutes; *Lower left:* 45 minutes; *Lower center:* 60 minutes; and *Lower right:* 90 minutes after injection. Frontal view.

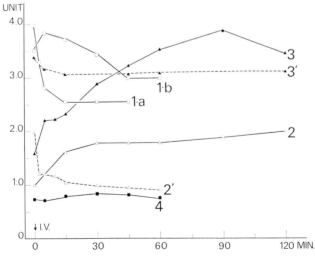

Fig. 86 Characteristic samples of uptake ratio patterns; **1-a.** Arteriovenous malformation. **1-b.** meningioma. **2.** Oligodendroglioma, astrocytoma and infarction. **2′.** An atypical example of oligodendroglioma (Fig. 85). **3.** Glioblastoma, carcinoma and sarcoma. **3′.** An unusual case of highly vascular carcinoma (Fig. 83). **4.** Intracerebral hematoma.

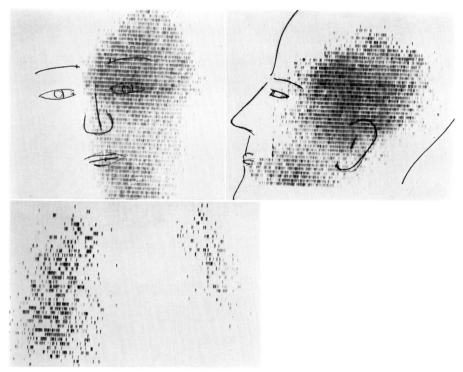

Fig. 87 [131]J MAA perfusion scan in a case of highly vascular sphenoid ridge meningioma. Common carotid injection. *Upper left:* frontal view and *Upper right:* left lateral view revealed high uptake in the tumor. Significant radioactivity in the lung (*Lower*) indicate the presence of arteriovenous fistula.

Brain abscess may not show the positive scan for a week or two after the onset of clinical symptoms. Also it is experienced that the scan remains positive for several months after the successful operation.

Demyelinating diseases, especially multiple sclerosis, may show the focal abnormality on the brain scan only during the period of exacerbation. In such an event, differentiation from the cerebral infarction seems to be impossible on the basis of the scan images alone.

7. "Doughnut" Sign in Brain Scanning

One peculiar pattern of radioisotope distribution may be seen in the positive brain scan, represented by a central core of relatively low radioactivity surrounded by a circular zone of higher activity. The picture is not unlike a doughnut, so that it has been named *"doughnut"* sign or *"halo"* effect in brain scanning (Figures 88–90).

Gottschalk and coworkers [45] seem to be the first to report this, and they noted this sign in eight of 80 positive brain scans (10 per cent). In our experience, however, the incidence is about three to four per cent of positive brain scans or 1 per cent of all cases [56], and O'Mara and coworkers [112] also reported an incidence of 2.9 per cent and 0.5 per cent, respectively.

The *"doughnut"* sign has been seen in many kinds of pathologies, and it is infrequent but non-specific. Metastatic carcinomas, glioblastomas, astrocytomas, oligodendro-

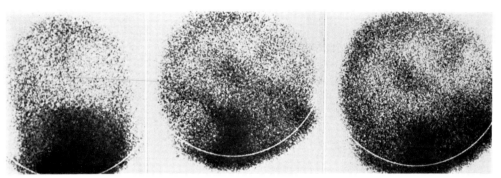

Fig. 88 Sarcoma of the brain. *Left:* Frontal view; *Center:* and *Right:* Right lateral views, one minute and five minutes after injection, respectively.

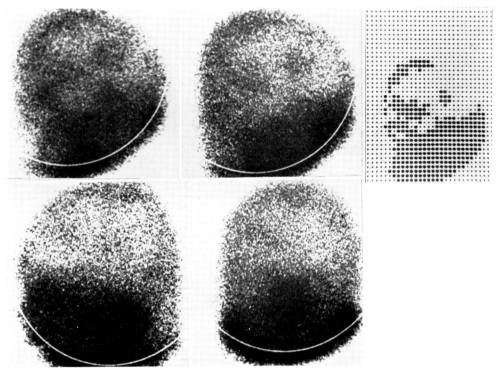

Fig. 89 Glioblastoma multiforme. *Upper left:* immediately after, *Upper center:* 15 minutes after, injection of ^{99m}Tc pertechnetate. Right lateral view. *Lower left:* Left lateral view. *Lower right:* Frontal view. *Upper right:* Map.

gliomas, cerebral infarctions, intracerebral hematomas, brain abscesses, encephalitic processes, and even meningiomas have been reported to be responsible.

In hematoma, infarction or abscess, the central portion of the lesion consists of the blood clot, necrotic brain tissue or pus, which is apparently poor in radionuclide accumulation. In the surrounding hyperemic and edematous tissue, on the other hand, radioactivity is high because of the reactive vascular changes or tissue edema, which causes the *"doughnut"* effect on external detection.

In most of the tumor cases in which the *"doughnut"* sign is reported, central necrosis or hemorrhage into the neoplastic tissue have been observed.

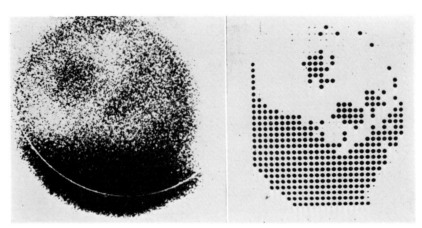

Fig. 90 Glioblastoma multiforme. Left lateral view. *Left:* ordinary scintigram; and *Right:* its map film.

Since the cystic formation or hemorrhage or necrosis in the central portion of the tumor is not rare, "*halo*" effect in the brain scan might be expected in more cases than are found in daily practice. However, the low activity in the central core is easily masked by the higher peripheral radioactivity so that the central cool area of small size may not be detected as such. In addition, the radionuclides diffuse slowly into the central necrotic region or into the cystic content and the scintigram in the delayed phase may show a homogeneous distribution of radioactivity. In fact, the "*doughnut*" sign is often found only in the early phase of sequential scintigraphy, and later study reveals a more or less homogeneous positive uptake of radioisotope in the whole area of the pathologic process, as shown in Figure 80.

Chapter XII

ROLE OF BRAIN SCANNING IN NEURORADIOLOGIC DIAGNOSTIC PROCEDURES

The well-taken history and the carefully performed general and neurologic examinations by well-informed, experienced neurologist or neurosurgeon are the most important agents for recognition and localization of brain tumors and other intracranial pathologies. It is true that there are no substitutes for them.

Brain scanning and other diagnostic technics—plain and laminographic roentgenograms of the skull, carotid and vertebral angiograms, air and positive contrast ventriculograms, cisternography and pneumoencephalography, echoencephalography, electroencephalography and thermography—, all provide useful adjuncts but none of them are perfect and each has its inherent shortcomings. Some of them are safe but less informative, others are not only unpleasant for the patients but also they are associated with a real risk of minor or serious complications. Some of the diagnostic technics are very informative for certain kinds of tumors but they are less useful for other kinds of diseases, and it is the great responsibility of the physician to assess the situation correctly and select the test which is most suitable for a given patient.

In the past, most brain tumor cases referred to the neurosurgeon showed bilateral choked discs and often blindness, dense hemiplegia and even coma, and the diagnosis of presence and the localization of the expanding mass was easy. Recently, however, the patient is referred to as a brain tumor suspect with a minor symptoms and signs, and the diagnosis tends to be much more difficult. Treatment of the brain tumor is, however, obviously much more successful when the tumor is still small and has not produced irreversible cerebral damage. In these early stages of the disease, history is often unrevealing and the general physical and neurologic examinations may be negative, and the diagnosis may have to depend largely upon the screening procedures with various diagnostic procedures.

Radioisotope brain scanning has the advantage that it can demonstrate the pathologic focus directly. Furthermore, it is absolutely safe, not unpleasant for the patient, and it can be performed repeatedly with various intervals in between. Recent advent of short-lived radionuclides and the development of imaging devices have enabled the examinations of a large number of cases within a short period of time. Thus it may well be expected that the radioisotope brain scanning will greatly help screening the patient even on an out-patient basis.

The relative value of brain scanning as compared with other diagnostic procedures has been studied widely [15, 17, 94, 124, 165]. Bucy and Ciric [17] compared the value of ^{99m}Tc pertechnetate brain scanning to other diagnostic tests in 100 brain tumor patients. Of their 100 patients reviewed, 26 were glioblastoma multiforme, 19 were metastatic lesions, 14 meningiomas, eight pituitary adenomas and craniopharyngiomas, eight astrocytomas, and six were diagnosed as acoustic neurinomas. The remaining 19 cases were various less common tumors such as epidermoid, oligodendroglioma, medulloblastoma and others.

Metastatic lesions were localized correctly by scanning in 89 per cent of cases, meningioma in 83 per cent and glioblastoma in 96 per cent. In comparison, the detection rate was 45 per cent to 55 per cent in astrocytomas and other gliomas of low grade malignancy, and was only 25 per cent in acoustic neurinomas, and the overall diagnostic accuracy fell to 67 per cent.

Diagnostic value of plain roentgenograms of the skull and electroencephalograms are summarized in Table 12. It has become obvious from this series that of these

Table 12 Diagnostic accuracy of clinical impression (history and neurologic examination), plain roentgenogram (per cent of abnormal findings), EEG (per cent of localizing EEG), and brain scanning (per cent of localizing scans) in 100 brain tumors (Bucy and Ciric[17])

Type of tumors	Clinical impression	Roentgenogram of skull	EEG	Brain scanning
Glioblastoma	81.8%	31.0	62.5	96.0
Astrocytoma	64.4	40.0	0.0	44.0
Other gliomas	66.6	33.3	—	55.0
Meningioma	64.4	66.6	25.0	83.2
Acoustic neurinoma	100.0	83.5	0.0	25.0
Pituitary adenoma and craniopharyngioma	88.8	100.0	—	0.0
Metastatic carcinoma	94.4	20.0	37.5	88.8
Total	80.4	43.2	25.0	67.0

procedures electroencephalogram is the least useful and least reliable for localizing purposes. Plain roentgenograms of the skull demonstrate one or more abnormalities in less than a half of cases and the radioisotopic brain scanning reveals focal abnormality in two thirds of cases as a whole.

However, more important than the diagnostic rate of each test for an entire group of cases is the fact that the relative values of various diagnostic tests differ widely from one kind of lesion to another, and this is clearly indicated also in our experience.

In our series of initial 101 cases of brain tumors, all were histologically verified except for 8 cases of deeply seated tumors in which the neuroradiologic contrast studies later confirmed the location of the expanding mass but the pathologic nature of the lesion could not be verified. The series includes 16 cases of meningiomas, 16 glioblastomas, 15 astrocytomas, 14 each of metastatic carcinomas and sellar-suprasellar tumors (craniopharyngiomas and pituitary adenomas), and five cases of acoustic neurinomas. As the screening test on an out-patient basis, only safe and not unpleasant procedures—plain roentgenogram of the skull, electroencephalogram, routine ophthalmologic examinations and ^{99m}Tc pertechnetate brain scanning—were selected.

Plain roentgenograms of the skull were interpreted as either *normal* or *abnormal*. Any changes compatible with the intracranial expanding mass, such as the separation of the suture line, increased digital markings, pathologic calcification, demineralization of the posterior clinoid process and dorsum sellae, shift of the calcified pineal body, and local bony destruction or hyperostotic changes were all classified as *abnormal*. Laminographies were not subjected to interpretation. Electroencephalograms also were classified into two groups, *normal* and *abnormal*.

As to the ophthalmologic examinations, each patient was subjected to fundoscopic examination and perimetry. Patient in whom the visual field defect, papilledema or optic atrophy was found in the absence of ocular diseases was categorized as *abnormal*. Brain scanning was classified as *abnormal* only when the focal accumulation of radioactivity was found definitely on two projections, and the equivocal scans were included into *normal* group. In this series of 101 cases, only the conventional scans at 15–30 minutes after administration of ^{99m}Tc pertechnetate were obtained and the sequential studies were rejected from the material. Interpretation of results of each study was done by the author, without knowing the clinical data or the results of other diagnostic tests.

The results are summarized in Table 13. Of 101 cases, plain roentgenograms of

Table 13 Diagnostic accuracy of several kinds of examinations. Number of positive results/Number of total examinations

Type of tumors	Number of cases	Skull films	EEG	Ophthal. exam.	Scan	All negative
Meningioma	16	8/16	6/10	10/16	14/16	0
Metastasis	14	4/14	4/6	5/13	13/14	1
Glioblastoma	16	7/16	5/7	15/16	14/16	0
Pituitary adenoma and craniopharyngioma	14	14/14	5/6	14/14	5/14	0
Acoustic neurinoma	5	4/5	1/2	5/5	3/5	0
Astrocytoma	15	6/15	5/6	7/13	10/15	0
Oligodendroglioma	3	1/3	0/0	3/3	3/3	0
Sarcoma	2	0/2	1/2	1/2	2/2	0
Ependymoma	4	1/4	3/3	3/4	3/4	0
Angioma	2	0/2	1/2	0/2	1/2	1
Malignant lymphoma	1	0/1	1/1	0/1	1/1	0
Deep, midline tumor	8	4/7	4/4	3/6	5/8	0
Pineal tumor	1	0/1	1/1	1/1	1/1	0
Total	101	100	50	96	101	*
No. Positive	*	49	37	67	75	*
% Positive	*	49	74	69	74	

the skull were available in 100, and one or more abnormalities were found in 49 (49 per cent positivity). Electroencephalography was performed less frequently, but in 74 per cent, or 37 of 50 cases, electroencephalograms were interpreted as *abnormal*. This high rate of abnormality of electroencephalogram looks incompatible with the 25 per cent positivity reported by Bucy and Ciric [17], however, their value of 25 per cent represents the *localizing* electroencephalographic abnormalities, whereas in our series all *abnormal* electroencephalograms were picked up irrespective of their localizing value. Detection rate of ^{99m}Tc pertechnetate brain scanning was 74 per cent, which compares favorably with the results of others.

The accuracy of each diagnostic test differed widely among the various kinds of

intracranial pathologies. In pituitary adenomas and craniopharyngiomas, plain roentgenograms of the skull revealed abnormality—enlarged sella turcica, sellar and suprasellar
calcification—in all of 14 cases and the nature of pathology was diagnosed correctly in
all of them. Fundoscopic examination and perimetry disclosed optic atrophy and/or
typical visual field defect in practically every case. In contrast, ^{99m}Tc pertechnetate
brain scanning was less revealing, it proved to be positive in only five of 14 cases
(36 per cent positivity). Electroencephalograms were abnormal in five of six cases
but in none of them they were of localizing value. In patients presenting with the
visual field defects and often with primary optic atrophy, plain skull roentgenography
apparently is the study of first choice and the ordinary brain scanning is less informative.

When metastatic carcinomas were considered as a group, plain roentgenograms of the
skull rarely showed the abnormality (four of 14 cases, or 29 per cent, in the present
series, or 20 per cent in the series of Bucy and Ciric [17]). When the pineal
gland is calcified, its shift across the midline may be of lateralizing value, but the
changes due to increased intracranial pressure are infrequent. On the other hand,
brain scanning proved to be positive in the high percentage of cases, 92 per cent in
this series, or 89 per cent in the series of Bucy and Ciric. It follows that, in the
patients suspected of harboring the intracranial metastatic tumor, particularly those
with a malignancy elsewhere in the body or the abnormal chest roentgenogram,
brain scanning apparently is the best diagnostic technic to begin with.

In our clinical series, two of four kinds of studies were performed in all of 101 cases and
in 96 cases three or all four studies were undertaken in combination. There were
only two out of 101 cases in whom all of two or three examinations failed to reveal
abnormality, one being a case of a small metastatic carcinoma and the other, an
angioma within the lateral ventricle.

From these results, it is evident that each of these diagnostic procedures is by no
means perfect and does not replace any of the others. When considered each technic
separately, there exist from 30–60 per cent false negatives. However, a combination of
some of these harmless tests actually improves the diagnostic accuracy and the purpose
of screening seems to be highly satisfied. There are large differences in the relative
value of each study according to the site and nature of the pathology, and the selection
of the best and most informative diagnostic procedure for each given patient—
the important task assigned to the clinician—is best helped by a careful history-
taking and examination of the patient.

In most clinical cases, a correct diagnosis as to the presence and localization of
brain tumor can be reached from the history, neurologic examinations, plain roentgenograms of the skull, electroencephalogram and brain scanning. In a few cases, resort
must be made to angiography, pneumoencephalography or to ventriculography and
other neuroradiologic contrast studies. These contrast studies are important also in
patients with known intracranial expanding lesions in order to further define their
location, nature, blood supply and impingement on the cerebral structures.

In Table 14, results of angiography, and/or air studies were correlated with those
of ^{99m}Tc pertechnetate brain scanning. Carotid and/or vertebral angiographies were
preformed in 93 out of 101 cases. The angiography was positive in localizing the
lesion in 87 cases, or in 95 per cent. Pneumoencephalography or pneumoventriculo-

Table 14 Diagnostic accuracy of several neuroradiologic examinations

	Angiography		Air study		Angiography and/or air study	
	Positive	Negative	Positive	Negative	Positive	Negative
Scan positive	66	5	35	2	70	2
Scan negative	21	1	15	2	22	0

graphy was done in 54 patients and proved to be positive in 50 cases (93 per cent positivity). Thus, the positivities of angiographies and air studies far exceed that of brain scanning. However, there were still six false negatives by angiography and four by air studies.

When the brain scanning was performed, seven of these 10 false negative cases were visualized directly and the false negatives in combined angiography-scanning series or air study-scanning series decreased to one and two cases respectively.

In 94 cases either angiography or air study or both were performed. There still remained two cases of false negatives, but both of them were correctly localized by brain scanning.

Similarly comparing cerebral angiography and brain scanning, Bucy and Ciric [17] also noted marked difference in their results among several kinds of tumors. In pituitary adenomas and craniopharyngiomas, or in acoustic neurinomas, angiography correctly localized the lesion in 75 per cent of cases, whereas the brain scanning was positive only in 25 per cent of cases in the former group and in none in the latter. On the other hand, in glioblastomas and in metastatic tumors, detection rate was higher by brain scanning than by angiography, although the differences were not large. Over-all accuracy of 79.1 per cent by angiography proved to be higher than 67.0 per cent value by brain scanning, but the difference seemed to be determined mostly by the number of basal tumors in the cerebellopontine angle or suprasellar-sellar region.

In the series of Rasmussen and coworkers [124], a total of 454 angiographic studies were performed in 501 patients with demonstrable pathologic processes. In about a half of the patients (52 per cent) there was noted displacement of either the anterior cerebral artery or the central vein or both. Dislocation of other vessels was noted in 58 per cent and in 32 per cent of cases abnormal vessels were seen, such as congenital vascular malformation, tumor vessels in malignant gliomas, tumor stain in meningiomas or cerebral metastases, or abnormal arterial inflow or venous outflow pattern in meningiomas or malignant gliomas.

Over-all accuracy was 72 per cent and 75 per cent for brain scanning and cerebral angiography, respectively. However, in only 59 per cent both studies were positive, and in 12 per cent both were negative, thus there was close agreement between the results obtained by the two methods in 71 per cent. Angiography was positive but scanning was negative in 16 per cent, conversely the brain scanning was positive but the angiography was negative in seven per cent and in the remaining six per cent scanning was positive but angiography was not definitely abnormal. In 13 per cent of cases, therefore, brain scanning proved to be superior to the cerebral angiography.

More important is the fact that the total accuracy was 80 per cent, in other words, diagnostic accuracy was increased by 16 per cent by cerebral angiography and 13 per cent by absolutely safe procedure of radioisotope scanning.

In the same series of Rasmussen and coworkers [124], pneumoencephalography was performed in 194 patients. Midline shift was noted in 39 per cent, impression of the ventricles in 48 per cent, ventricular dilatation in 20 per cent, and poor filling or dislocation of the infratentorial structures in 10 per cent. When the pneumographic findings were matched with the scanning results, both tests were positive in 39 per cent and both were negative in 16 per cent, that is there was close agreement between the results obtained by two methods in 55 per cent of cases. Positive pneumographic study with negative brain scanning was noted in 29 per cent, and the reverse was true in 11 per cent. In the remaining five per cent, brain scanning was positive but the pneumography was inconclusive. Over-all detection rates were 68 per cent for pneumography and 55 per cent for scanning. The two studies combined had an accuracy of 84 per cent. Therefore, it is evident that pneumoencephalography increased the accuracy of localization by 29 per cent and brain scanning by 16 per cent.

All these data clearly indicate that, although the over-all accuracy of brain scanning does not reach the level of angiography or air study, brain scanning, when combined with those contrast studies, does provide useful adjunctive data and reduces the false negatives markedly. This is particularly important since the brain scanning is easily performed, not unpleasant to the patient and practically without morbidity even in the infant, the aged, or the severely-ill patient.

Chapter XIII

PERFUSION BRAIN SCANNING AND DETECTION OF ARTERIOVENOUS FISTULA WITH ^{131}I MAA

1. [131]I MAA Perfusion Brain Scanning

When injected into the artery, macroaggregates of human serum albumin measuring 10 μ or more are filtered out by capillaries. If the aggregates are labeled with the radioactive tracer, the rate of accumulation of radioactivity in the target organ can be externally collimated, and this is expected to be directly proportional to the blood flow destined for that particular organ.

The method has been widely used for the study of the pulmonary circulation. It was applied to the brain for the first time by Kennady and Taplin [73] in 1965. They injected ^{131}I MAA (10–100 μ in diameter) into the internal carotid artery of the monkey, and found no detectable central nervous system abnormalities with the doses below 2.0 mg protein. They concluded that the initial arteriolar entrapment of the macroaggregates appeared to be purely a physical mechanism.

King, Wood and Morley [75] in 1966 reported the use of ^{131}I MAA in clinical brain scanning. Complications were noted in four of 12 patients, and in two of them, complications (focal seizures in one and right hemiplegia and aphasia in the other) occurred in close association with the injection of the macroaggregates. They advised caution in the clinical use of this material.

On the other hand, Rosenthall, Aguayo and Stratford [133] reported their experience of 50 ^{131}I MAA brain scans in 42 patients. Carotid injections were performed 43 times and vertebral injections were done seven times. A transient reduction in amplitude in the occipital leads of electroencephalography was noted in one case following vertebral injection, but this patient had exhibited similar changes with a prior injection of normal saline. Otherwise, no deleterious effect was encountered, and the pathologic studies of the brain in six patients, who later came to necropsy, revealed no changes attributable to the injection of the ^{131}I MAA.

Since that time, several papers on ^{131}I MAA perfusion scanning of the brain have appeared, and the intracarotid injection of the material has been recognized to be a safe and often valuable adjunctive method of scanning [32, 33, 107, 132, 145]. In our experience of more than 100 carotid injections and several cases of vertebral injections, a syncopal attack of short duration has been encountered once, but no other complications have ever been met [50].

In evaluating the macroaggregates perfusion brain scans, we must identify the position of the needle tip. When the needle is introduced into the internal carotid

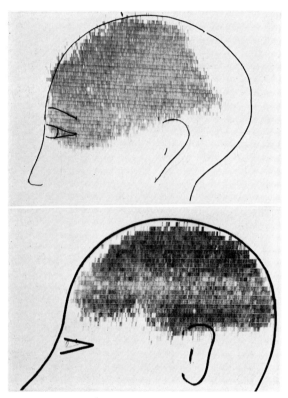

Fig. 91 Perfusion scan in normal subject, left lateral view following internal carotid injection. *Upper:* anterior and middle cerebral arterial territories are filled; *Lower:* posterior cerebral territory is filled in addition.

artery (Figure 91), the distribution of radioactivity is limited to the cerebral hemisphere and the orbital contents. The territory of the middle cerebral artery is visualized constantly, and the area of the anterior cerebral artery in most of the cases. In addition, the territory of the posterior cerebral artery is filled in 20–30 per cent of cases in which the posterior cereceral artery is of carotid origin. If the needle tip is placed in the common carotid artery, a considerable portion of the radioactive tracer is lost to the external carotid artery (Figure 92), and in the lateral view the posterior cranial fossa stands out in the scintigram as an area of low background activity. Injection into the external carotid artery may present a scintigram more or less similar to that following common carotid injection, but the heavy deposit of the radionuclide in the maxillar region enables the differentiation from the latter occasion.

Secondly, the time lapse between the injection and scanning is important since the macroaggregates disappear from the capillary bed rather rapidly, a false diagnosis of ischemic lesion may be reached if the scanning is delayed. According to Briz-Kanafani and Lazos-Constantino [12], this may happen especially in the temporal lobe where the disappearance of the macroaggregates is more rapid.

Thirdly, it should be borne in mind that the cold or ischemic zone does not necessarily indicate a primary lesion, since the direct or indirect pressure on the arteries due to the tumor itself or the herniation of the brain, may result in the similar changes.

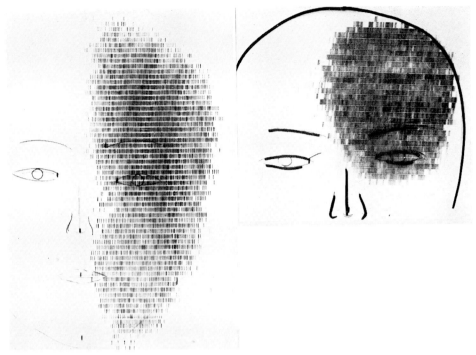

Fig. 92 Perfusion scan in normal subjects. *Left:* common carotid injection; *Right:* internal carotid injection, bilateral anterior cerebral arteries are filled.

In general, lateral view is more useful than the frontal view since, in the latter, the thickness of the brain to be scanned is much greater.

The diagnostic significance of macroaggregates perfusion scanning does not seem to have been fully evaluated. In 1969, Briz-Kanafani and Lazos-Constantino [12] reported their experience in 50 cases. Of the 50 patients, the procedure was considered to be effective and the result positive in 40 (80 per cent). In five patients (10 per cent) the scans could not be read because of error in position of the needle. In the remaining five (10 per cent) scan image could not be correlated with the clinical lesion and was classified as negative.

Later in 1970, the same authors [13] reported on 24 patients who underwent autopsy from one day to eight months after the macroaggregates perfusion scanning. The histopathologic study in each case suggested that the macroaggregates were innocuous and that they did not obstruct small vessels in any permanent sense. Of the total of 24 patients there was clear and evident correlation between the perfusion brain scan and the autopsy finding in 17, and in the remaining seven patients anatomic lesion had produced no change in the perfusion scan, or the scan depicted only the secondary change at a distance from the true lesion. In 12 of a total of 24 cases the anatomic diagnosis was that of primary neoplasm and in eight of them there was a positive correlation between the perfusion scan and the anatomic lesion. In seven cases of cerebrovascular disease, correlation was better, positive correlation being obtained in six.

Dietz and coworkers [32] reported that the positive results were obtained in 70 per cent of all tumor cases, the value much the same as that of ^{99m}Tc pertechnetate brain scanning (74 per cent positivity).

Huber and Rösler [69] detailed their experience in 126 patients in whom both the macroaggregates perfusion scanning and the angiography were carried out. Of 42 patients with angiographically localized tumors, perfusion scanning was positive in 33 (78.6 per cent), and negative in nine (21.4 per cent). Cerebrovascular diseases were diagnosed in 30, in 22 of them (73.4 per cent), the macroaggregates perfusion scanning was also successful in localizing the lesion and in eight cases of chronic subdural hematoma, intracerebral hematoma or contusion with edema of the brain, perfusion scanning was positive but one.

In 27 cases in which angiograms were interpreted normal, perfusion scanning revealed a cool focus in three. In one of them, subcortical hematoma was found, in one cerebrovascular accident was diagnosed and in the remaining one the cool focus on the perfusion scan seemed to represent the site of negative exploration for neoplasm. In a further 19 cases suspected of harboring the intracranial space-occupying lesion or cerebrovascular accidents, perfusion brain scanning revealed a cool focus in 13 and a focal increase in radioactivity in three. In eight of these 19 cases, the localization of the lesion could be made only with a combination of angiography and perfusion brain scanning.

From these results, Huber and Rösler reached the conclusion that "angiography provides more accurate information than the angioscintigraphy (macroaggregates perfusion scanning) in most cases, especially on the nature of the pathologic process," but that "combination of the two methods can be useful in cases where angiography alone fails to afford precise information," with which our experiences are in absolute consonant.

Positive results in perfusion brain scanning may be presented either as a cool focus or a hot focus. Usually the cool focus means that the pathologic lesion has much less radioactivities than in the surrounding brain, because of the scanty development of the capillary beds in the lesion or the focal ischemia due to vascular occlusion. Occasionally, however, there are arteriovenous fistulas in the pathologic sites so that the macroaggregates may not be trapped within the lesion but passed freely through the arteriovenous short-circuits into the venous side of the circulation. In this occasion, the scanning of the lung easily reveals the presence of arteriovenous shunts in the territory of the artery injected with the macroaggregates (Figure 93).

Pathologic processes which demonstrate the cool focus in the macroaggregates perfusion scans include any kind of cystic tumor, abscesses, hematomas, anemic infarctions and cerebral contusions or edema, and as the lesion with arteriovenous fistulas the arteriovenous malformations and malignant gliomas may be added to the list (Figures 94 and 95). Extracerebral masses which compress the brain but are not perfused by the injected carotid artery, such as the extracerebral hematomas, and the tumors of the skull and the meninges, above all the meningiomas also show the focal decrease in radioactivity in the perfusion brain scanning. Of particular importance is the metastatic carcinoma of the brain, which is often surrounded by severe reactive edema. Even when the metastatic deposits are still quite small and undetectable by the conventional scanning, a large area of decreased radioactivity in the perfusion scan, representing the peritumoral edema, may be quite helpful in the detection of the metastatic deposits (Figure 95, left).

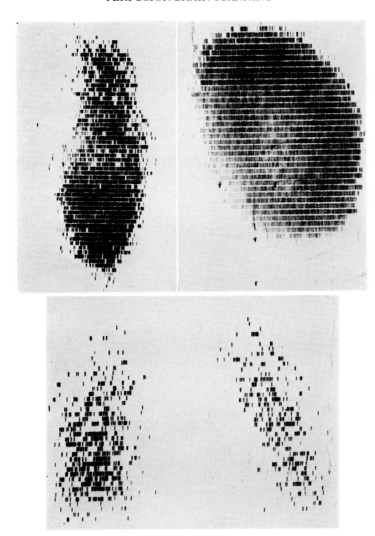

Fig. 93 Perfusion brain scan in arteriovenous malformation in the left frontal region. *Upper left:* and *Lower:* frontal view and pulmonary scan following left common carotid injection, showing the presence of arteriovenous fistula; *Upper right:* internal carotid injection after operation. Perfusion of brain is improved. No significant radioactivity in the lung.

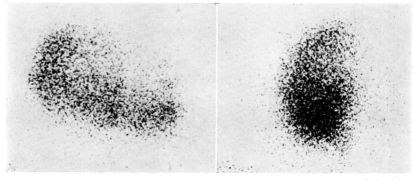

Fig. 94 Perfusion brain scan in glioblastoma multiforme in right frontal lobe. *Left:* right lateral view after internal carotid injection; *Right:* frontal view.

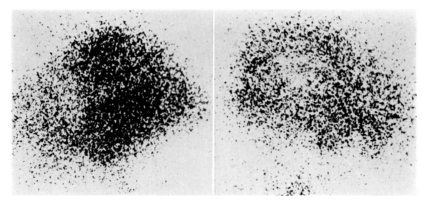

Fig. 95 Perfusion brain scan. *Left:* left lateral view in metastatic carcinoma in left frontal lobe; *Right:* right lateral view in intracerebral hematoma.

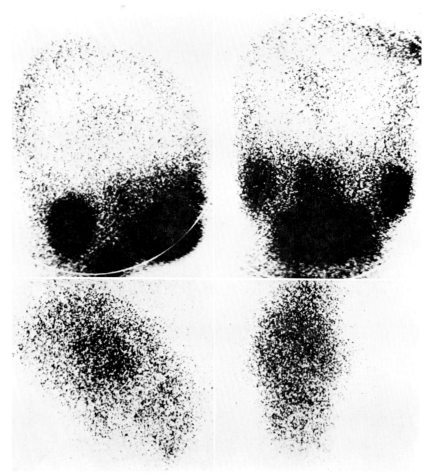

Fig. 96 Highly vascular oligodendroglioma. *Upper left:* Right lateral and *Upper right:* frontal view of ^{99m}Tc pertechnetate scintigram; *Lowe left:* Right lateral and *Upper right:* frontal view of perfusion brain scan.

The lesion which demonstrates the hot focus on the macroaggregates perfusion brain scans suggests the pathologic process which is rich in vascularity without any significant arteriovenous short-circuits, such as some kinds of gliomas, cerebral infarctions with rich collateral circulation, or meningioma when the feeding artery is injected with the tracer agent (Figure 96).

Practically, the cool type of focus far outnumbers the hot type of lesion in the perfusion brain scanning. In the series of Huber and Rösler, 26 of 33 positive scans in the tumor cases, 20 of 22 with cerebrovascular accidents, and seven of eight in traumatic conditions presented the focus of reduced radioactivity. Thus, of 80 cases 63 were diagnosed by the perfusion brain scanning and in 53 of them (84.1 per cent) the focus proved to be cool.

It is concluded from the results quoted above and from our personal experiences that the perfusion brain scanning with the macroaggregates is a useful adjunctive method of localizing the organic lesions in the brain as well as the extracerebral space-occupying lesions, and provides us with a useful information of the pattern of cerebral circulation. It is especially informative in the diagnosis of lesions of ischemic nature.

The procedure seems to be safe and innocuous. However, the catheterization of the large arteries in the neck is obligatory for this purposes, and this is evidently a drawback inherent to the procedure. As long as the carotid or the vertebral artery is once catheterized, the arteriography generally yields far more abundant and accurate information both on the localization and the nature of the lesion. Our policy at the present time is to carry out the perfusion scanning only in cases where the angiography is not conclusive, and the macroaggregates injection is made through the same catheter or needle used for the preceding angiography in an attempt at avoidance of multiple punctures of the artery. Moreover, in the recent cases, ^{133}Xe scanning or ^{99m}Tc pertechnetate angiography is being performed instead of the macroaggregates perfusion scanning, although the scintigram tends to be more blurred in ^{133}Xe scan than in the macroaggregates perfusion scan because of the gradual diffusion of xenon gas into the ischemic focus, and the arteriovenous shunt can not be detected by xenon scanning, either.

Section scanning after intra-arterial injection of the radioiodinated macroaggregates, or the computer display of the scan data, is expected to enhance the accuracy of the perfusion scanning, and these methods seem to be a significant armamentarium not only for the diagnosis of cerebral lesions, but also for the reseach studies on the cerebral circulation.

2. Detection and Quantification of Arteriovenous Fistula

When there exists a sizable arteriovenous fistula in the territory of the artery injected, significant amounts of the macroaggregates are not filtered by the capillary bed but they pass freely through the arteriovenous short-circuits into the venous side, and they are eventually trapped by the capillary bed of the lung. Therefore, combined brain and lung scans may be expected to help detecting the direct arteriovenous communications in the cerebral vasculature.

Practically, the use of macroaggregates in the study of an arteriovenous short-circuits in the local circulation has been recorded in several organs. Ueda and coworkers [152], as early as in 1965, reported the successful external detection of a portocaval shunt by means of a lung scan following the injection of ^{131}I MAA directly

into the spleen. Rosenthall, Aguayo and Stratford [133] also described the positive
lung scans in the case of an angioma of the brain after intracarotid injection of
^{131}I MAA.

In our experiences in cases with arteriovenous malformation, carotid-cavernous sinus
fistula or malignant glioma or meningioma with an overt vascular stain and arteriovenous
short-circuits demonstrated by angiography, the procedure of macroaggregates brain-
lung scanning was a safe and effective measure for detecting and semiquantitating the size
of the arteriovenous fistula. Pre- and postoperative studies were performed and the
effect of surgery, namely eradication of the fistula and the improvement of cerebral
circulation could be easily determined. Reports of several illustrative cases follow.

Figure 97 shows a case of an arteriovenous malformation in the right temporo-
occipital region. Preceding carotid angiography revealed that both the external and
internal carotid arteries fed the arteriovenous anomaly, and the vascularization of the
brain was very poor. The needle catheter was first introduced into the right external
carotid artery and 100 μCi of ^{131}I MAA injected. Brain scanning showed radioactivities
limited to the maxillar and thyroid regions. A large portion of the macroaggregates
passed into the lung (Figure 97, left). A few days later, the internal carotid artery
was punctured and ^{131}I MAA injected. Radioactivity in the brain was restricted to the

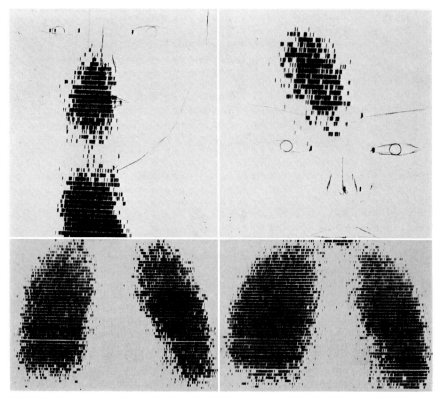

Fig. 97 Arteriovenous malformation in the right temporo-occipital region, supplied by external
and internal carotid arteries. *Left:* right external carotid injection; *Right:* right internal
carotid injection. Marked radioactivity in the lung demonstrates presence of large
arteriovenous shunts in the lesion.

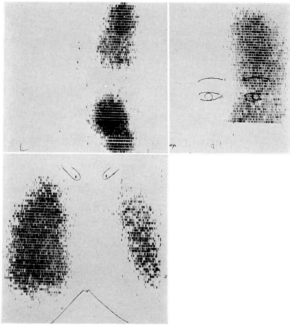

Fig. 98   Arteriovenous malformation. *Left:* Preoperative, left common carotid injection; *Right:* after complete removal of the lesion, left common carotid injection. No radioactivity in the lung.

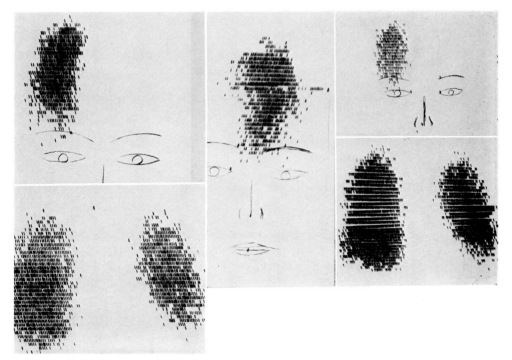

Fig. 99   Carotid-cavernous fistula, right. *Left:* brain and lung scan. Right internal carotid injection indicates the presence of arteriovenous shunt; *Center:* after left internal carotid injection. No radioactivity in the lung; *Right:* after incomplete occlusion of the right common carotid artery. Increase in the shunt rate is shown by enhanced radioisotope accumulation in the lung as compared to the preoperative result.

small area of the frontal lobe, instead, most of the macroaggregates were seen in the lung (Figure 97, right).

Figure 98 represents the records of an another case of cerebral arteriovenous malformation. Brain scanning after injection of the macroaggregates into the left common carotid artery showed the radioactivity in the maxillar region and in the territory of the middle cerebral artery but not of the anterior cerebral artery in the brain. Accumulation of high radioactivity in the lung clearly showed the presence of arteriovenous fistula (Figure 98, left).

At surgery an arteriovenous malformation was totally extirpated. The left anterior cerebral artery which was not visualized on the preoperative angiogram was nicely filled postoperatively. On repeat macroaggregates brain-lung scans, the macroaggregates were injected again into the left common carotid artery, but the radioactivity in the lung did not exceed the level of the background activity. Brain scan, however, showed the diffuse distribution of the radioactivity in the brain and the face, and the territory of the anterior cerebral artery was well shown (Figure 98, right). Comparison of the pre- and postoperative scans thus demonstrates the disappearance of the fistula and the improvement in perfusion of the brain.

Figures 99 and 100 show the pre- and postoperative studies in two cases of carotid-cavernous sinus fistula. In Figure 99, internal carotid injection of macroaggregates

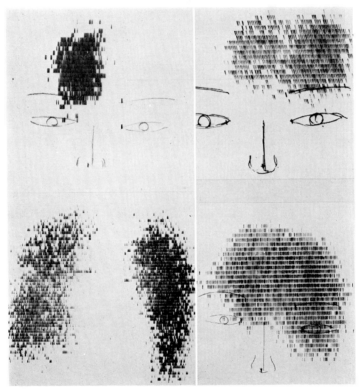

Fig. 100 Carotid-cavernous fistula, right side. *Left:* preoperative, right internal carotid injection demonstrates the presence of arteriovenous shunt; *Upper right,* preoperative, left internal carotid injection with right carotid compression; No radioactivity in the lung; *Lower Right:* after trapping the fistula. Left internal carotid injection shows no radioactivity in the lung.

showed the presence of a large arteriovenous shunt on the right side (Figure 99, left). Injection of the macroaggregates into the left internal carotid artery with the manual compression of the right carotid showed the distribution of radioactivity in the territories of the left middle and bilateral anterior cerebral arteries but no activity in excess of the background was noted in the lung (Figure 99, center). This was in agreement with the left carotid angiogram, which showed the filling of both anterior cerebral arteries but not of the fistula. After trapping of the fistulous opening, the repeat injection of the macroaggregates into the left internal carotid artery revealed the radioactivity limited to the brain (Figure 99, right).

Figure 100 is the records of the case of spontaneous carotid-cavernous sinus fistula on the right side. Again in this case, the fistula was fed from the right internal carotid artery (Figure 100, left), but not from the left (Figure 100, upper right). As the patient could not tolerate the total occlusion, the right common carotid artery was partially ligated in the neck. Bruits and proptosis persisted. Repeat brain-lung scanning revealed that the short-circuiting of the macroaggregates injected into the right carotid artery was increased (Figure 100, lower right).

Naturally, no quantitative estimation is possible with regard to the size of the fistula by this procedure. We used to classify the brain-lung scans arbitrarily into three categories; "*negative*" when no activity in excess of the background is noted in the lung scan; "*one plus*" when the pulmonary scan is less dense than that of the brain; and "*two plus*" when the density of the lung scan is the same as, or greater than that of the brain; and the results in general seem to be in good agreement with the angiographic and clinical findings of the patients [50]. Although the angiographies, especially serial angiographic studies which provide morphologic information such as the type, size and location of the lesion and the anatomy of the feeding and draining vessels are indispensable for the diagnosis of cerebral arteriovenous fistulas, the macroaggregates scanning provides us with the information not only about the presence and the approximate size of the fistula but also about the perfusion of the brain at the capillary level, and this procedure evidently is a valuable adjunctive method in the study of cerebral arteriovenous fistulas.

We tried to estimate the size of the fistula semiquantitatively [51]. For this purpose, a scintillation detector is positioned over the right or left upper quandrant of the chest of the patient lying supine on the table. Thirty-five to 50 μCi of ^{131}I MAA is injected into the carotid or the vertebral artery and the count rates were monitored continuously. After 10 to 15 minutes the same dose of ^{131}I MAA is given into the vein and the recording repeated without changing the position of the detector.

Shunt rate:

$$\frac{\text{Volume of Flow Shunted through the A.-V. Fistula}}{\text{Total Flow of Carotid or Vertebral Artery Injected}}$$

is determined as follows:

$$\text{Shunt rate} = \frac{a}{b} \times \frac{B}{A} \times 100 \text{ (per cent)}$$

where a = count rates after intra-arterial injection (height of plateau, or "a" in Figure 101, A); b = count rates after intravenous injection (height of plateau, or "b" in Figure 101, B); A = net counts of ^{131}I MAA administered intra-arterially; and B = net counts of ^{131}I MAA injected into the vein (Figure 101).

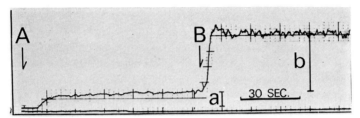

Fig. 101   A: intra-arterial injection, B: intravenous injection.

$$\text{Shunt Rate} = \frac{a}{b} \times \frac{B}{A} \times 100 \text{ (per cent)}$$

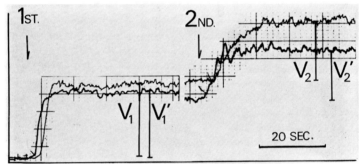

Fig. 102   Repeat intravenous injections.
V_1 and V_2, counts over the right lung;
V_{1}' and V_{2}', counts over the left lung.

$$\frac{V_1}{V_2} = \frac{V_1'}{V_2'}$$

In several healthy subjects, two intravenous injections of ^{131}I MAA were carried out consecutively and the count rates over the chest were monitored. Although the absolute count rates differed widely between the two injections, the count rates corrected for the net counts of ^{131}I MAA injected showed no significant variations.

In several other normal subjects or fistulous patients, two detectors were placed over each side of the chest and intra-arterial and intravenous injections of macroaggregates were performed. "Shunt rate" calculated separately for each side did not show any significant difference. On the basis of these preliminary results, the technic seems to be reproducible(Figure 102).

The calculated "shunt rate" for the internal carotid injection in 8 healthy volunteers ranged from 18.9–22.0 per cent, the average being 20.3 per cent (S.D. = ±1.4).

The mean value of 20.3 per cent in the "shunt rate" in healthy subjects needs brief comment. The presence of the precapillary "throughfare channels" and rarely in the white matter of the brain, short unbranched arteriovenous anastomoses up to 25 μ in diameter, have been reported in the literature [59]. It does not follow, however, that such channels are quantitatively significant so as to permit the short-circuiting of up to one-fifth of the internal carotid artery flow in the normal subjects.

The macroaggregates of radioiodinated human serum albumin which we used in the present study are reportedly uniform in size (20–100 μ) and contain only a minimum number of free iodine molecules, but, it seems possible that a certain number of smaller-sized particles passed freely through the vascular bed of the brain, and in addition it has been actually observed under the microscope that the macroaggregates once trapped in the vessels measuring 15–25 μ in diameter are eventually swept forward by the pulsatile flow of blood plasma and formed blood elements. Regional vasodilatation has also been reported to occur in the small vessels distally to the temporary occlusion, triggered probably by the acidosis of the tissue rendered ischemic. Thus it seems quite reasonable to assume that a portion of the macroaggregates, initially entrapped in the capillary bed of the brain, can eventually clear the vascular filter and pass to the lung.

Whatever the seeming shunt rate of 20.3 per cent in the normal subjects implies, important is the fact that the calculated values in normal subjects are rather constant with only a minimum individual variation. In practice, the results of application of the procedure in the fistulous patients were satisfactory, and in all cases where the arteriovenous fistulas were present, the calculated shunt rate significantly exceeded the control value of 20.3 per cent. The technic proved to be a sensitive investigative method for detecting even the slightest degree of short-circuiting, and the over-all results were in good agreement with the clinical and angiogrpahic findings (Table 15).

Table 15 Shunt rates in 11 cases of cerebral arteriovenous fistulas. AVM; arteriovenous malformation, CCF: carotid-cavernous sinus fistula, ICA; internal carotid artery, ECA; external carotid artery, VA; vertebral artery

Case no.	Diagnosis	Artery injected	Shunt rate (%)	Remarks
2	AVM, lt.	lt. ICA	93.1	
8	CCF, lt.	lt. ICA	36.7	Study #1
		lt. ICA	55.4	#2
		rt. ICA	39.6	#2
		rt. ICA	41.5	#2, with compression of lt. carotid
13	AVM, lt.	rt. ICA	58.8	
		lt. ICA	92.9	
14	AVM, lt.	rt. ICA	38.0	
		lt. ICA	42.0	
15	CCF, rt.	rt. ICA	82.0	
		lt. ICA	28.6	
16	AVM, posterior fossa	lt. VA	32.3	
17	AVM, rt.	rt. ICA	41.8	
		rt. ECA	21.2	
18	AVM, rt.	rt. ICA	69.1	
19	AVM, rt.	rt. ICA	26.5	
		lt. ICA	22.1	
20	AVM, lt.	lt. ICA	42.1	
21	AVM, lt.	lt. ICA	50.8	

A representative case is shown of a patient with the carotid-cavernous sinus fistula on the left side, which was filled from the internal carotid artery on both sides. The shunt rate following left internal carotid injection of the macroaggregates was 36.7 per cent in the first examination. In the following week the patient complained of an increase in her ptosis and the bruits, and the repeat angiography also proved the entlargement of the fistula and the poor filling of the cerebral arteries. At this time, the

Table 16   Changes in shunt rates by functional test

Case no.	Shunt rate (%)	
	Control	After breath-holding
2	93.1	97.5
9	27.8	32.2
18	39.8	51.2
21	50.8	56.3
	Control	Following papaverine
9	27.8	20.6
10	69.5	60.3
20	42.1	35.3
21	50.8	37.5
	Control	Hyperventilation
18	39.8	51.2

shunt rate also increased from 36.7 per cent to 55.4 per cent. In this patient, the shunt rate following right internal carotid injection was 39.6 per cent which did not change significantly with the manual compression of the left carotid artery in the neck.

In several cases, tests were repeated during breath-holding, hyperventilation or after the intracarotid injection of papaverine hydrochloride. Although the studies were performed in the limited number of cases, an increase in the shunt rate during breath-holding or hyperventilation, and a decrease following administration of papaverine was noted (Table 16).

Such a functional test in shunt rate determination is expected to enhance our knowledge of hemodynamics of cerebral arteriovenous fistulas.

Chapter XIV

RADIONUCLIDE CEREBRAL ANGIOGRAPHY

The use of near-ideal radioisotope such as ^{99m}Tc pertechnetate with a gamma ray scintillation camera permits the visualization and delineation of vascular structures. This is accomplished by performing rapid sequential scintiphotography while the radioisotope bolus traverses the cerebral vascular structures. Such studies as called radionuclide angiography or the first stage study of serial scintiphotography have proved to be the method of rapid and safe approach in the assessment of cerebrovascular diseases and vascular characterization of various other intracranial lesions [129, 131].

For this purpose, a large dose of ^{99m}Tc pertechnetate or another comparable short-lived radionuclide is injected rapidly, either intravenously or intra-arterially. We have used 10–15 mCi of ^{99m}Tc pertechnetate in most cases, but recently several studies were performed with 10 mCi of ^{169}Yb DTPA.

On most occasions, radionuclide is injected rapidly into the antecubital vein as a bolus, and rapid serial three or four second exposures are obtained manually on the Polaroid film or with the Nikon motor drive and a 35-mm high speed black-and-white film.

When the studies are carried out immediately following the contrast angiography, radioxenon brain scanning or rCBF determinations, injection may be made into the artery through the same catheter as used for the previous study. Exposure time is shortened to one to two seconds when the injection is made intra-arterially.

Frontal view is the routine for intravenous radionuclide angiography, whereas the lateral view is preferred for the intra-arterial study or when the lateralization of the lesion is clinically evident. In all cases, the radionuclide angiography is followed by standard or conventional scintiphotography.

On eight to 12 second exposure scintigram of an intravenous cerebral ^{99m}Tc pertechnetate flow study in a normal subject, radioactivity is noted in the paramedian portions of the neck, representing the carotid arteries on both sides. Usually 12–16 second exposure scintigram shows a symmetrical right and left blush and the midline radioactivities, the former corresponds to the middle cerebral arterial tree and the latter to the anterior cerebral artery.

Already at 16–20 seconds, the superior sagittal sinus begins to be depicted as a midline radioactivity, and the high radioactivity may be noted in the region of the transverse sinus and trocular Herophili on 16–20 or 20–24 second exposure film (Figure 103).

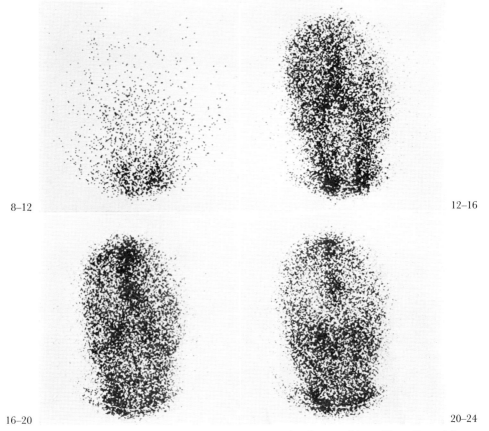

8–12   12–16

16–20   20–24

Fig. 103   Intravenous radionuclide angiography. Frontal view in a healthy subject. From left to
right, 8–12, 12–16, 16–20 and 20–24 second exposures after intravenous injection of
10 mCi of ^{99m}Tc pertechnetate.

In the aged, arteriosclerotic, or the patient with congestive heart failure, the arrival of
radionuclide is delayed by several seconds in accordance with the prolongation of the
arm-to-retina circulation time, and the inflow pattern of radioisotope becomes more
insidious so that the arterial blushes often fail to stand out clearly on the scintigram.

Addition of radionuclide angiography to the conventional scintigraphy enables us to
make a gross assessment of the perfusion of the brain.   The significance of radionuclide
angiography in cerebrovascular occlusive disease and in cerebral arteriovenous malformations has been discussed.

Serial imaging during the initial passage of the radioisotope bolus through the
cerebral vasculature allows one for the detection of intracranial lesions not yet associated
with blood-brain-barrier abnormalities detectable by the conventional scanning.   Subdural hematoma of recent onset, chronic cystic lesions and gliomas of low grade
malignancy, which tend to escape detection by conventional method, can be detected
by this means [37].   Recently, it has been reported that the brain death can be defined correctly with radionuclide angiography [43].

Figure 104 illustrates a right lateral view of intra-arterial radionuclide angiography
in a case of middle cerebral artery occlusion. ^{99m}Tc pertechnetate in dosis of 10 mCi

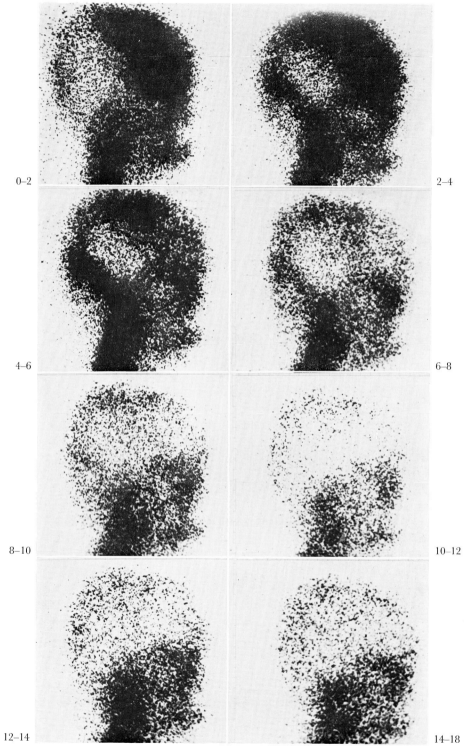

0–2

2–4

4–6

6–8

8–10

10–12

12–14

14–18

Fig. 104 Right middle cerebral artery occlusion. Intra-arterial ^{99m}Tc pertechnetate angiography, two-second exposure serial films, right lateral view.

was injected into the right common carotid artery through the catheter used for the preceding carotid angiography, and the rapid serial two-second exposure scintigrams were obtained.

On 0 to two second exposure scintigram, the territory of the anterior cerebral artery was filled with radioisotope, but the middle cerebral area was entirely devoid of radioactivity. On two to four second exposure, the superior sagittal sinus, torcular Herophili and the transverse sinus started to become filled and on four to six second exposure, further washout of the radioactivity in the anterior cerebral territory and the denser radioactivity in the transverse sinus were well shown. The area of supply of the middle cerebral artery remained cool throughout the course of radionuclide angiography.

Figure 105 is the left lateral view of the same patient as in Figure 104. On this side, carotid angiography revealed that the internal carotid artery was completely occluded immediately distal to the ophthalmic artery and the cerebral arteries were partly filled by way of the transdural cortical anastomoses via the hypertrophied ophthalmic artery, middle meningeal artery, superficial temporal artery and the occipital artery.

Ten mCi of ^{99m}Tc pertechnetate were injected into the common carotid artery and the two-second exposure serial films were obtained. On 0 to two second exposure scintigram, the territory of the external carotid artery was well filled but the area of the brain was entirely cool. The occipital, superficial temporal and the middle meningeal arteries were prominent. Single branch of the internal carotid artery, the ophthalmic artery, was seen as a radioactive blush, which represents the important collateral role of this artery. Also found on this film is the irregular shaped, rather dense, radioactive area over the superior posterior frontal region, which persisted onto the four to six second exposure scintigram. When compared with the preceding angiogram, this corresponds clearly to the arterial network of transdural anastomoses between the cerebral arteries and the middle meningeal-superficial temporal group.

Another case of carotid occlusion is illustrated in Figure 106. The patient presented with abrupt onset of hemiplegia on the right side. Carotid angiography demonstrated a total occlusion of the internal carotid artery distal to the ophthalmic artery, and the transdural internal carotid-external carotid anastomoses were found in the posterior superior frontal region as well as in the temporal region, the latter one being exceptionally prominent like a network of medium-sized vessels.

^{99m}Tc pertechnetate in dosis of 10 mCi was injected into the common carotid artery and two second exposure serial scintigraphy was performed. Scintigram showed the distribution of radioactivity in the areas of the external carotid artery. A round, dense radioisotope accumulation was found in the retroauricular area, and another blurred and irregular shaped focus in the superior frontal region. Both of them corresponded apparently to the sites of well developed collaterals by way of transdural anastomotic channels.

In this case and several other cases of carotid artery occlusion, remarkably increased radioactivity was noted in the nasopharyngeal area. Mishkin and Dyken [103] reported that in 17 out of 900 radionuclide angiograms obtained with ^{99m}Tc pertechnetate, the nasal area contained marked radioactivity prior to or coincidental with the activity in the major cerebral arteries. All but one showed anatomical or functional occlusion of one or both internal carotid arteries with a patent external carotid artery. Contrast angiography demonstrated obstruction of one internal carotid artery in 11 and obstruction of both internal carotid arteries in one, while brain

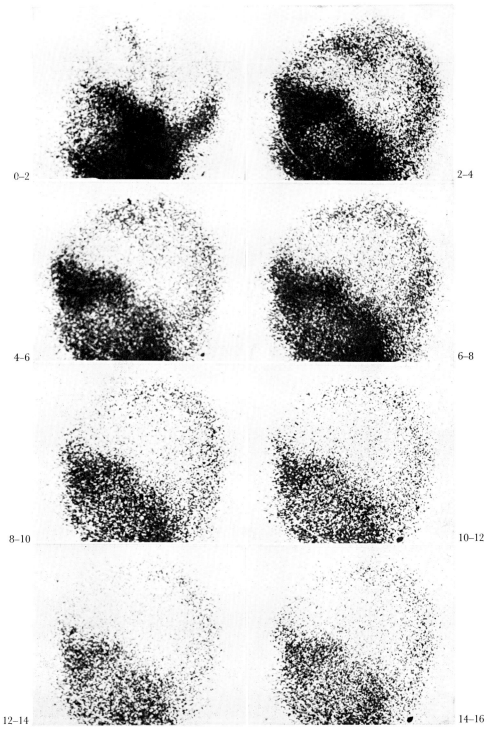

0–2

2–4

4–6

6–8

8–10

10–12

12–14

14–16

Fig. 105 Left internal carotid occlusion. Intra-arterial ^{99m}Tc pertechnetate angiography, two-second exposure serial films, left lateral view.

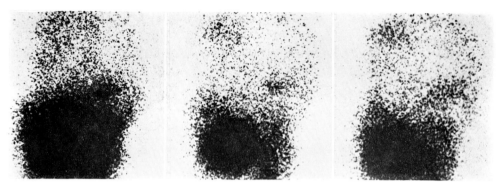

Fig. 106 Left internal carotid occlusion. Intra-arterial two-second exposure radionuclide angiograms, left lateral view.

death was diagnosed in four. Only three cases with proven internal carotid artery
occlusion failed to display the increased radioactivity in the nasopharyngeal area,
or "hot nose" sign.

The external carotid artery serves as an alternate and important route of blood
flow to the brain when the internal carotid artery is obstructed. Since the degree of
collateral development of various available routes differs greatly between the individuals,
inequality of activity in certain areas of normal external carotid arteries is the rule, as
seen in Figures 105 and 106.

Normally, activity in the nasal area becomes apparent when the venous sinuses and
jugular veins contain the radioactivity. When the internal carotid artery becomes
occluded, increased blood flow through the external carotid artery may cause an increase in radioactivity also in the nasopharyngeal area during the early arterial phase
prior to filling of the sagittal sinus. This early increased radioactivity seems to
cause "hot nose," which has been seen to occur within 24 hours after occlusion.

The experiences of Mishkin and Dyken [103] and of ours indicate that a "hot nose"
on radionuclide angiogram should strongly indicate the functional (non-filling due to
increased intracranial pressure) or anatomical occlusion of the internal carotid artery.

Figure 107 illustrates a right lateral view of rapid serial scintigraphy in a patient
presented with a choked disc and a left hemiparesis. On 0 to two second exposure, there
was noted extremely intense radioactivity in the territory of the middle cerebral artery.
The territory of the anterior cerebral artery was almost completely cool. On the two to
four second exposure film, the posterior portion of the superior sagittal sinus, torcular
Herophili and the transverse sinus were already filled. The radioactivity in the
middle cerebral territory was still intense and the area of the anterior cerebral
artery displayed the parenchymatous phase of the radionuclide angiography. On
four to six second exposure film and later, concentration of radioactivity in the center
of the hemisphere decreased significantly but it still remained high. Conventional
scintigram taken two minutes after injection showed a high, round uptake in the fron-
toparietal region.

Carotid angiogram in this patient showed a round tumor with prominent tumor
vascularity and the early filling of veins draining into the superior sagittal sinus.
Histology of the tumor was a glioblastoma multiforme.

Another example of glioblastoma multiforme is illustrated in Figure 108. In this

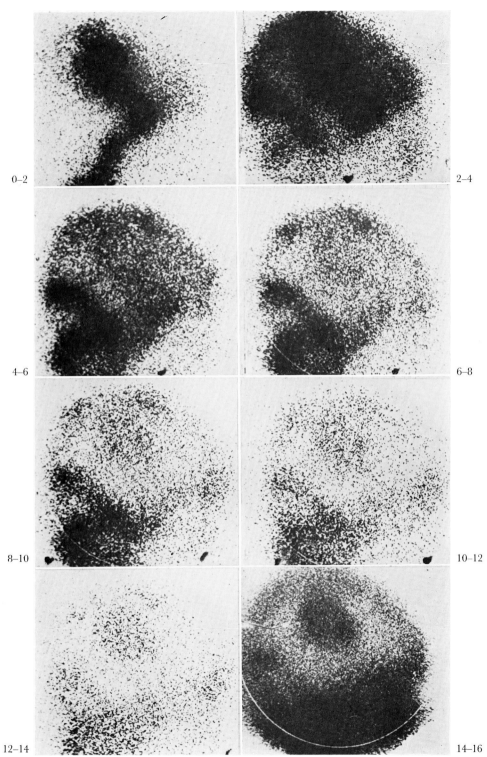

0–2

2–4

4–6

6–8

8–10

10–12

12–14

14–16

Fig. 107 Glioblastoma multiforme in the right parietal region, two-second exposures, right lateral view, and conventional scintigram two minutes later.

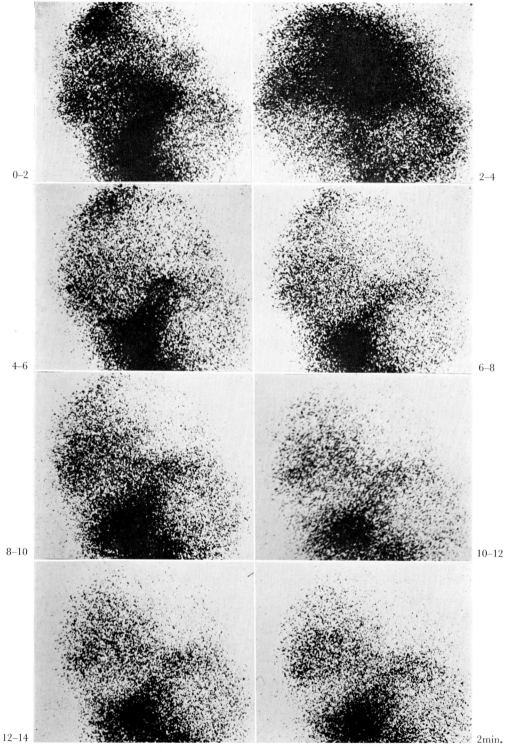

0–2

2–4

4–6

6–8

8–10

10–12

12–14

2min.

Fig. 108 Glioblastoma multiforme in the right cerebral hemisphere. Intra-arterial two-second exposure films, right lateral view.

patient, a partial resection of right parietal glioblastoma with occipital lobectomy was performed and ^{60}Co irradiation was combined with intravenous vincristine therapy postoperatively.

A few months later, the symptoms and signs of increased intracranial pressure recurred and the clinical course was downhill thereafter. Preceding carotid angiography revealed diffuse involvement of the right parieto-temporo-occipital lobes with the recurrent tumor, but no distinct tumor stain or abnormal vessels were found. Radionuclide angiography disclosed inequal and irregular distribution of the radioactivity over the right cerebral hemisphere on the initial two or three films of the serial studies. Later series of radionuclide angiography and a conventional scintigram revealed increased radionuclide accumulation in the right parietal, temporal and occipital regions.

In a case of glomus jugulare tumor, the increased and early accumulation of radioactivity was noted on the first few films of intravenous radionuclide angiography (Figure 109). Conventional scintigrams were entirely negative including the vertex, posterior and angled posterior view. In this case, therefore, the pathology might have escaped detection if the rapid serial scintigraphy was not performed as a routine procedure in brain scanning.

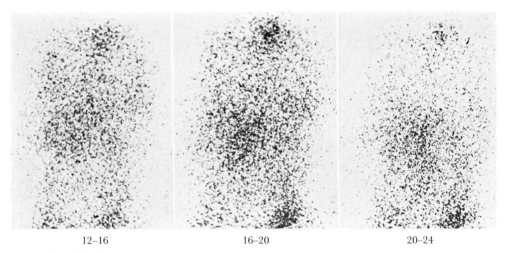

12–16   16–20   20–24

Fig. 109 Right glomus jugulare tumor. Intravenous four-second exposure frontal views.

Since most of the radionuclide apparently remains in the blood during the initial passage of the bolus through the cerebral vasculature, the lesion with increased vascularity is often best depicted by intracarotid or intravenous radionuclide angiography. The purely vascular lesions such as the arteriovenous malformations or giant aneurysms of the cerebral arteries are the best examples, but many neoplastic lesions can produce a vivid focus on the radionuclide angiogram. Highly vascularized glioblastoma is often seen to produce a hot focus on the radionuclide angiogram. Then the focus becomes once blurred, however, it again increases in radioactivity with the progressive accumulation of radioisotope in the tumor tissue.

In Figure 110, a case of cavernoma of the cavernous sinus is shown. In this patient carotid and vertebral angiographies revealed a huge mass in the left middle

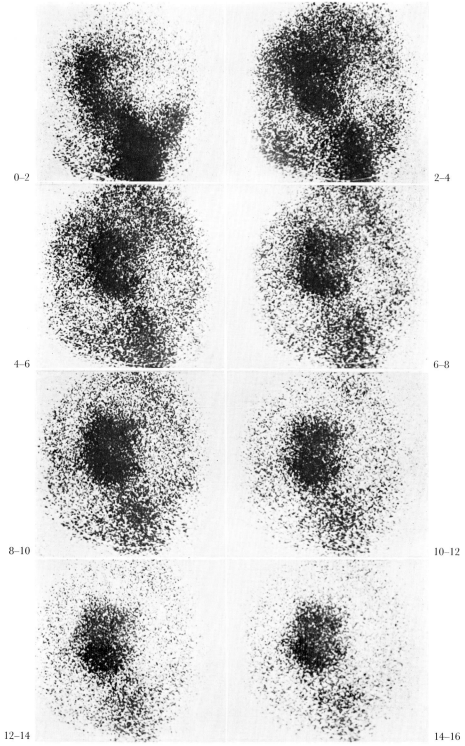

0–2
2–4
4–6
6–8
8–10
10–12
12–14
14–16

Fig. 110 Cavernoma of cavernous sinus, left. Intra-arterial two-second exposure radionuclide
angiograms, left lateral view.

fossa. Anterior peripheral zone of lesion showed sparse tumor vessels supplied from the internal carotid artery, and the faint tumor stain at the posterior limit was fed by the vertebral artery. Radionuclide angiography was performed following the carotid angiography, the injection of 10 mCi of ^{99m}Tc pertechnetate being performed via the catheter placed into the common carotid artery. On 0 to two second exposure, carotid artery in the neck and the occipital branch of the external carotid artery was shown as blush. In addition, there was noted an intense, sickle-shaped radioactivities in the anterior temporal region. On two to four second exposure film, the region of the anterior and middle cerebral arteries were filled. On the later films, abnormal radioactivity of the tumor changed its shape gradually—the posterior portion of the tumor became filled and the initially filled anterior portion faded— and finally, on 12–14 and 14–16 second exposures there was found a round, rather homogeneous accumulation of radioactivity. In this case, the simultaneous storage and display of the transit data of ^{99m}Tc pertechnetate showed greatly prolonged circulation time within the tumor. rCBF determination by ^{133}Xe found that the tumor blood flow was generally equal to that of the brain.

Cavernoma of the brain is composed of dilated, numerous vessels and contain huge amounts of blood. Its removal often causes prohibitive bleeding. On angiogram,

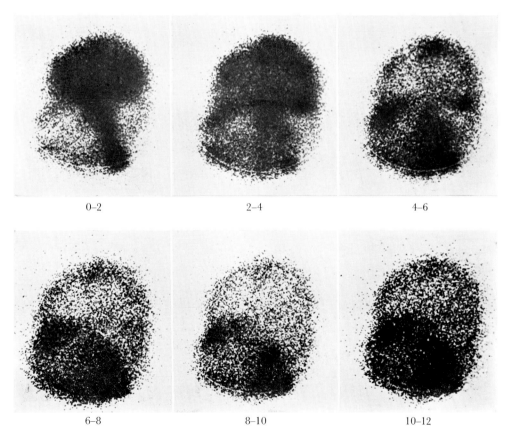

0–2   2–4   4–6

6–8   8–10   10–12

Fig. 111 Oligodendroglioma, left. Intra-arterial three-second exposure radionuclide angiograms, left lateral view.

however, it has been reported that the visualization of intense tumor stain or dilated feeding arteries is rare. Such angiographic and operative characteristics were true in the present case. Radionuclide angiography and radioxenon brain scanning, combined with the transit time study and the rCBF determinations, suggest that the tumor contains a large blood pool, but that the circulation in the tumor vasculature is extremely retarded so that the blood flow remains not enhanced. These radioisotopic data seem to clarify the discrepancy between the tissue vascularity as proved by

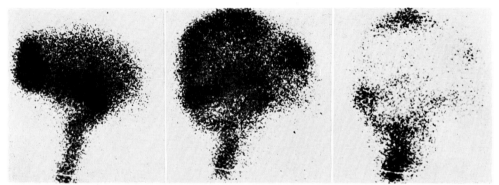

Fig. 112 Right occipital arteriovenous malformation. Intra-arterial injection, two-second exposures, right lateral view.

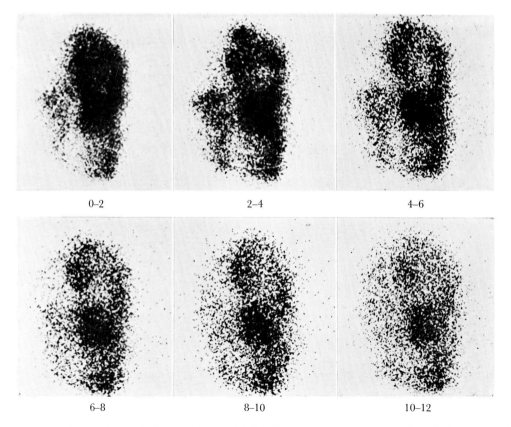

Fig. 113 Falx meningioma. Intra-arterial injection, two-second exposures, frontal view.

operation and histology, and the poor demonstration of tumor stain on angiogram.

Figure 111 illustrates the lateral view of radionuclide angiography in a case of oligodendroglioma involving the frontal lobe on the left side. Clinically, the patient presented the papilledema, generalized convulsions and a slight dysphasia. Carotid angiography disclosed the displacement of vessels compatible with the large, infiltrating tumor in the left frontal region, but no tumor stain or abnormal vessels were found.

Following angiography, radionuclide angiography was performed with 10 mCi of ^{99m}Tc pertechnetate injected into the left common carotid artery. On 0 to two second exposure, the distribution of radioactivity appears rather homogeneous but on two to four second and four to six second exposures, focal increase in radioactivity in the parietal parasagittal area and diffuse area of reduced radioactivity in the frontal lobe are noted. The conventional scintigrams taken later however were normal throughout the sequential studies up to one hour after injection.

Comparing the radionuclide angiography with the carotid angiography, the focal high radioactivity in the parietal area was interpreted to represent the large veins. Low radioactivity in the whole frontal lobe conformed well to the angiographic features of diffuse avascular mass, and the diagnosis of glioma of low grade malignancy was made, which was subsequently proved at operation.

Several other cases which showed the early increased radioactivity on the radionuclide angiography were illustrated in Figures 112 through 114.

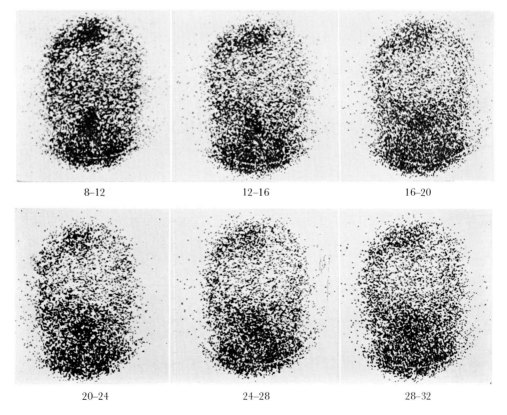

| 8–12 | 12–16 | 16–20 |
| 20–24 | 24–28 | 28–32 |

Fig. 114 Right parasagittal meningioma, intravenous injection, four-second exposures, frontal view.

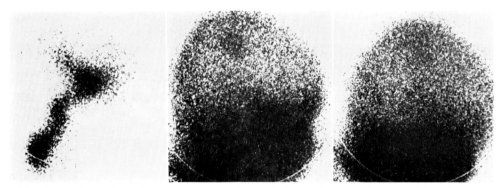

Fig. 115   Metastatic carcinoma, right parietal. *Left:* 0–2 second exposure intra-arterial angiogram; *Center:* Conventional scintigram at one minutes after injection; *Right:* Scintigram at 30 minutes postinjection.   Right lateral view.

Cystic tumor, glioma of low grade malignancy, hematoma, peritumoral gliotic tissue or edematous brain can be revealed as an area of localized poor perfusion on radionuclide angiography.

Figure 115 is a composite of radionuclide angiography and conventional scintigram in a case of metastatic carcinoma in the right parietal lobe.   On 0 to two and two to four second exposures, there was noted a large area of low perfusion in the right cerebral

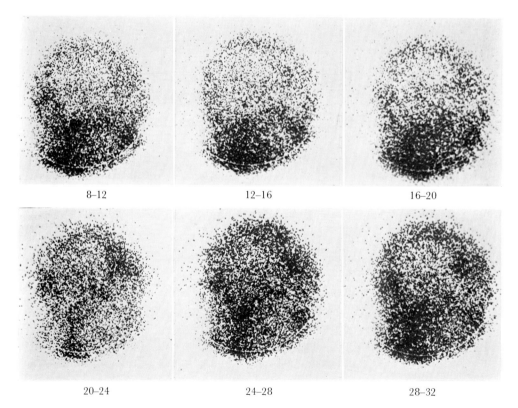

8–12   12–16   16–20

20–24   24–28   28–32

Fig. 116   Right frontal glioblastoma multiforme. Intravenous injection, four-second exposures, right lateral view.

hemisphere. Conventional scintigram 2 minutes after injection revealed a round uptake with a blurred margin in the parietal region, which faded rapidly. Angiography showed a feature suggesting a large frontal mass.

Combined radionuclide angiography and contrast angiography seemed to indicate a solid and rather vascular tumor in the parietal lobe associated with a cyst in the frontal lobe. At operation, the metastatic nodule was found in the subcortical region of the parietal lobe, accompanied by an intense swelling and partial necrotic liquefaction of the frontal lobe.

Although the radionuclide angiography by intra-arterial injection has been described in some detail in the present chapter, intra-arterial injection was limitedly used in the cases where the studies were done immediately after the contrast angiography. Several illustrative cases of intravenous radionuclide angiography are shown in Figures 116 through 119.

As a part of routine sequential brain scanning, intravenous radionuclide angiography was done mostly with the detector placed for the anterior view. By doing this, symmetry of the hemispherical perfusion could be compared easily and was confirmed further by a transit time study.

In the series of Rosenthall and Martin [135], about 45 per cent of patients with acute cerebrovascular occlusive disease had a reduced perfusion or radioactivity on the

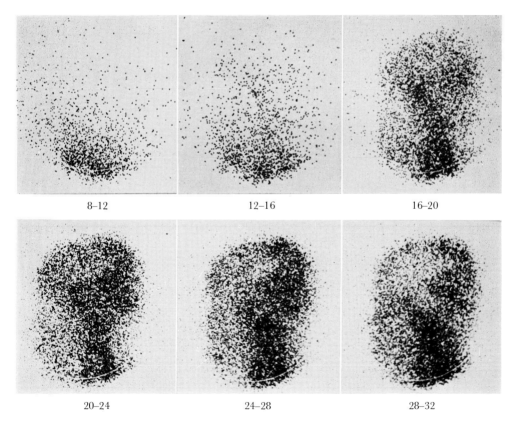

| 8–12 | 12–16 | 16–20 |
| 20–24 | 24–28 | 28–32 |

Fig. 117 Left convexity meningioma in the occipital region. Intravenous injection, four-second exposures, left lateral view.

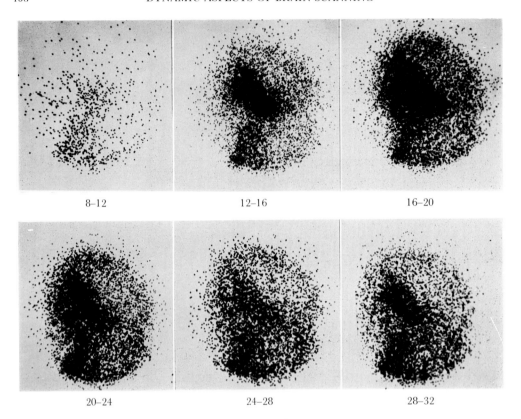

8–12   12–16   16–20

20–24   24–28   28–32

Fig. 118 Right occipital arteriovenous malformation. Intravenous injection, four-second exposures, right lateral view.

affected side, and 30 per cent demonstrated this difference when the static images were negative. The combined use of radioactivity transit study yielded a detection rate of 57 per cent, which is an improvement of 54 per cent over the incidence of a positive static image. Eight out of 22 patients (37 per cent) with the clinical transient cerebral ischemia had a reduced perfusion on the side of the insult. In all of these cases the study was performed at the time of symptomatology, but this high yield of abnormal transit study seems to be rewarding.

In the category of the intracranial neoplasm, the perfusion of the radioactive tracer may be rich and rapid, or conversely low and delayed on the side of involvement. Generally in the metastatic tumor, higher perfusion on the side of the lesion is rare, probably due to the association of peritumoral edema.

In the glioma of low grade malignancy and the cystic tumors, the perfusion of the involved hemisphere tends to be delayed and decreased.

On the other hand, in the highly malignant gliomas, higher radioactive transit is often seen on the side of the lesion. Although this conforms well to the visualization of the abnormal tumor vessels associated with the early filling of veins and implies a vascular nature of the neoplasm, it should be realized that the cerebrovascular occlusive disease may rarely demonstrate higher radioisotope transit on the side of the lesion, probably as a manifestation of "luxury perfusion" around the lesion.

In the traumatic cases, Rosenthall and Martin noted a higher incidence of dissimilar

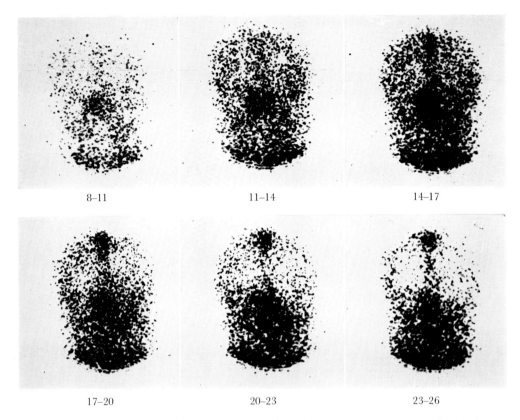

8–11   11–14   14–17

17–20   20–23   23–26

Fig. 119 Carcinoma of frontal sinus. Intravenous injection, three-second exposures, frontal view.

perfusion in the case of contusion than in concussion.   Two of three subdural hematomas showed a reduced transit of the radioactivity on the involved side.

In a group of 20 patients with cerebral atrophy, five (25 per cent) had dissociation of hemispheric radioactive transit, but the parallel relationship could not be found between the perfusion abnormality and the electroencephalographic findings. They also found a similar incidence of unequal radioactivity transits in patients with psychiatric conditions and in groups of patients with metabolic and nutritional disturbances of the brain.

In hydrocephalus, the displaced middle cerebral arteries and veins could be found as the depression and lateral deviation with decreased width of the middle cerebral blush in the frontal view of radionuclide angiography [69].   Generalized increase in cerebral circulation has been experienced by Rössler and Huber [130] and by us in hyperthyroidism, and nonfilling of the cerebral vessels have been confirmed by radioisotope transit study in brain death cases.   We have also found in a few cases the retention of the radioactivity over the injected hemisphere, when the radionuclide angiography was carried out immediately following contrast angiography.   Repeat study one week later found bilaterally symmetrical perfusion.   Although this is an rare experience, it might mislead the diagnosis.

Radionuclide angiography has been proved to yield valuable information as to the vascular characterization of the brain in cerebrovascular disease, primary and secondary cerebral neoplasms, traumatic cases, and in several other occasions. This procedure, particularly the intravenous one, is entirely safe and harmless to the patient. The intra-arterial method provides more accurate information and as far as being done following the contrast angiography using the same needle it does not add to the morbidity to the patients.

Now it is our routine to start the brain scanning with the radionuclide angiography and to obtain the sequential scintigrams up to one or two hours after injection. This has improved the scan results considerably, and when combined with the recording and graphic display of the radioisotope transit data, diagnostic accuracy of brain scanning is expected to further increase.

Chapter XV

BRAIN SCANNING AND QUANTIFICATION OF CEREBRAL BLOOD FLOW BY USE OF A SCINTILLATION CAMERA AND [133]XENON

The use of a short-lived radionuclide ^{133}Xe as an agent for scanning has been made possible by rapid imaging with a scintillation camera. When injected into the artery, washout of ^{133}Xe is proportional to the regional blood flow and the pattern of sequential images during the intra-arterial injection and of desaturation depicts the differences in blood content and blood flow in the perfusion area of the artery involved [54, 55, 134]. It is assumed that the visualization of vascular patterns of the brain may provide a useful information on the diagnostic as well as the therapeutic problems.

More recently, the combined use of a 1,600 channel multiparameter analyzer, magnetic tape system, printer, and more recently the data-store/playback accessory equipped with the video-tape recording unit has enabled the quantification of regional cerebral blood flow, in addition [54, 55, 58, 61, 62].

For the purpose of ^{133}Xe brain scanning and cerebral blood flow study, the patient is placed supine and the gamma-ray scintillation camera is set to image either the frontal or lateral view of the head. [133]Xe in doses of three to seven mCi dissolved in 10 ml of physiologic saline is injected into the carotid artery through a Teflon catheter needle either over a 30 second period or rapidly in two to three seconds.

For the purpose of sequential scintigraphy, eight serial exposures on the Polaroid films are obtained manually at the speed of one for each 30 second period. In addition, a 35 mm film is exposed at the speed of one frame for each 30 second period covering a whole period of 10 to 18 minutes after injection. Data storage and retrieval can be carried out by the use of a video-tape system.

In case of cerebral blood flow study, the scintillation camera with a 4,000 hole collimator is used for registration. Three methods are available for the study.

1) After the intracarotid injection of ^{133}Xe in normal saline, radioactivity of the brain is sampled in one half of the $12^1/_2$ NaI crystal of the scintillation camera connected to a rate meter and a potentiometer plotter, and the washout curves obtained are analyzed.

2) The scintillation camera is combined with a 1,600 channel memory, dual analog-to-digital converter, data processor, oscilloscope, high speed parallel printer and a computer compatible magnetic tape system. Impulses from the scintillation

camera are localized in the 1,600 matrices of 40 by 40, and stored in the magnetic tape for 10 minutes.

Total count rates for each matrix for the first 15 seconds and those for the entire 10 minutes are printed out and the blood flow indices are calculated arbitrarily as follows:

$$\text{Flow Index (FI)} = \frac{\text{Total Counts for the First 15 Seconds}}{\text{Total Counts for the Entire 10 Minutes}}$$

Flow indices calculated separately for each of 1,600 channels are rearranged on a section paper with 40 by 40 matrices and the blood flow index map (FI-Map) is obtained.

Reviewing the FI-Map, the regions of interest (ROIs) consisting of the selected four (two by two), six (two by three), or nine (three by three) channels are selected for further study. Playing back the tape into the 1,600 channel memory, count rates for each record are printed out. Using these data, washout curves are drawn and the compartmental analyses are performed.

3) More recently, information from the scintillation camera is fed directly into the data-store/playback accessory. After the examination is over, the magnetic tape is replayed and the washout curves are drawn directly with dual-pen recorder. This method has advantages over the previous ones in that the ROIs of the desired size, shape and location can be selected.

1. Brain Scanning with ^{133}Xe

When ^{133}Xe dissolved in the normal saline is injected into the internal carotid

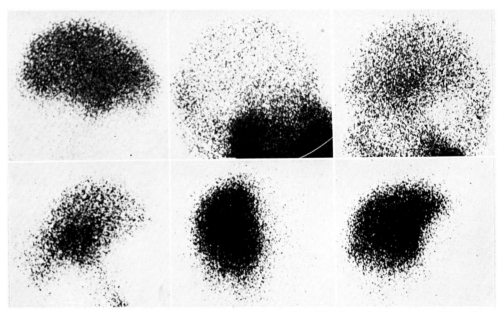

Fig. 120 ^{133}Xe brain scan in normal subject. *Upper left:* right lateral view, internal carotid injection; *Upper center:* right lateral view, external carotid injection; *Upper right:* left lateral view, common carotid injection; *Lower left:* left lateral view, internal carotid injection, anterior cerebral territory not filled; *Lower center:* frontal view, right internal carotid injection; *Lower right:* frontal view, right internal carotid injection, radioisotope distribution crossing the midline.

artery, the scintigram depicts the territories of the anterior and middle cerebral arteries, and occasionally of the posterior cerebral artery when it arises from the internal carotid artery.

The common carotid injection demonstrates both the internal and external carotid territories, sparing the area of supply of the vertebro-basilar system. When injection is made selectively into the external carotid artery, the scintigram at first glance is not unlike that of common carotid injection, but the radioactivity in the facial region is markedly high when compared to that in the brain (Figure 120).

From our experience it seems that the territory of the artery injected as well as the anatomical and physiological patterns of blood flow through the major cerebral arteries can be detected by means of ^{133}Xe brain scanning, but the abnormality in the flow pattern of the second order branch of the cerebral artery can not be assessed with any certainty.

Pathological ^{133}Xe brain scans are classified into two main types. (Table 17) In the Type 1, the lesion is characterized by a focal increase and/or rapid clearance of the radioactivity. The lesion appears hot during the injection period, thereafter, it tends to become rapidly homogeneous, or rather cool. In some cases, the scintigram shows homogeneous distribution of radioactivity and no increase in accumulation of the tracer is noted initially. After this, however, the pathologic focus becomes progressively cold and the later films clearly demonstrate a circumscribed focus with decreased radioactivity.

Table 17   Two types of radioxenon brain scans

TYPE 1 FOCUS:
   Factor: Increase in blood flow and/or blood pool in the focus.
   Xenon scan:
   Initially   Later
      Hot————————————→ Homogeneous
      Homogeneous————————→ Cold
   Pathology encountered: Arteriovenous malformation, angioma, meningioma, malignant glioma, etc.

TYPE 2 FOCUS:
   Factor: Decrease in blood flow and/or blood pool in the focus.
   Xenon scan:
   Initially   Later
      Homogeneous————————→ Hot
      Cool————————————→ Homogeneous
   Pathology encountered: Cyst, hematoma, benign glioma, infarction, etc.

This type of focus is found in arteriovenous anomalies, angiomas, and malignant gliomas. Some cases of meningioma also showed this pattern as long as the ^{133}Xe was injected into the feeding arteries (Figures 121 and 122).

Initial high radioactivity associated with rapid clearance in this type of lesion shows that the focus is rich in blood content and/or blood flow, and this was invariably proved by angiographic demonstration of tumor vasculature, by a regressive course of ^{99m}Tc pertechnetate uptake in the sequential brain scanning, and finally by the operative and histologic findings.

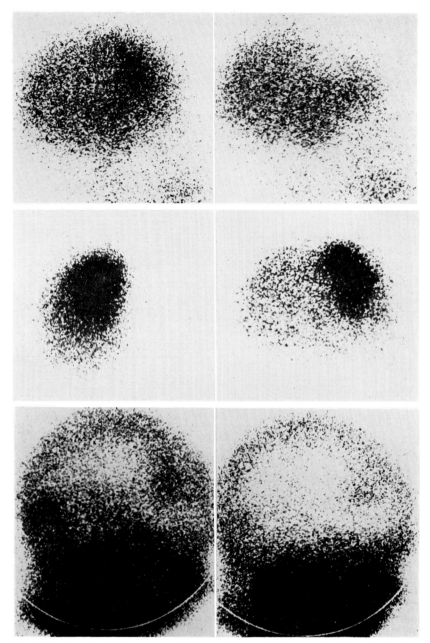

Fig. 121 Right frontal glioblastoma multiforme. *Upper:* 0–30 second (*left*) and 45–75 second (*right*) exposure ^{133}Xe scans, right lateral view; *Middle:* ^{131}I MAA perfusion scan, frontal view (*left*) and trigh lateral (*right*) view. *Lower:* ^{99m}Tc pertechnetate scan. Immediately after (*left*) and 10 minutes after (*right*) administration of ^{99m}Tc pertechnetate, right lateral view.

On the other hand, when the blood flow is reduced in the pathologic focus as in Type 2 lesion, a decrease in the radioactivity is slower in the focus than in the normal brain. During the injection period, the size of the blood pool in the lesion affects the scintigraphic picture, in addition. This second type of ^{133}Xe scintigrams were obtained

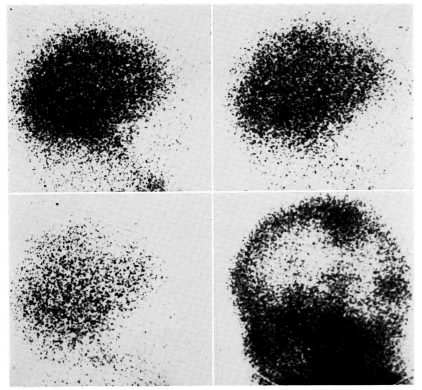

Fig. 122 Meningioma, left parietal region. *Upper left and right, and Lower left:* 30 second exposure ^{133}Xe scan, left lateral view; *Lower right:* ^{99m}Tc pertechnetate scan, left lateral view.

mainly in the cystic tumor, hematoma, glioma of low grade malignancy, peritumoral edema and cerebral infarction, all of which were shown as avascular space-taking mass at operation and histologic study also demonstrated poorly vascularized lesion (Figures 123, 124, and 125).

When the ^{133}Xe brain scanning is performed for the diagnostic purposes, it provides useful adjunctive informations mostly in Type 2 lesions, in which the ^{99m}Tc pertechnetate scanning is not infrequently negative or equivocal, and the angiographic study shows the presence of an avascular mass but its size and extent are difficult to estimate because of lack of vascular stains.

However, it should be pointed out that the ^{133}Xe brain scanning needs the puncture of the carotid artery, which is by no means absolutely free of morbidity. We consider the indication for the study rather strictly, and as far as possible, the study is performed immediately following the angiography using the same needle catheter and avoiding renewed multiple carotid artery punctures.

It should also be noted that, when monitored externally with a gamma-ray scintillation camera, a certain level of difference in the blood content or blood flow volume must be reached before the focus stands out clearly against the background radioactivity. In addition, the margin of the focus tends to be ill-defined with time, and the cold focus in ^{133}Xe brain scanning tends to be smaller than ^{131}I-MAA perfusion scan

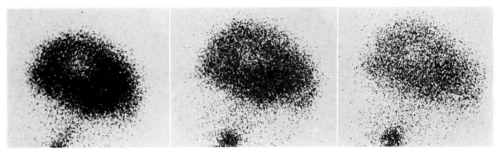

Fig. 123 Intracerebral hematoma. From *Left* to *Right:* 30 second exposure ^{133}Xe scan, left lateral view.

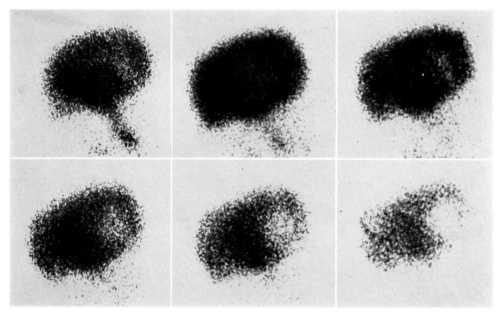

Fig. 124 Left occipital convexity meningioma. From *Upper left* to *Lower right:* 30 second exposure ^{133}Xe scans, internal carotid injection, left lateral view.

images or than the actual size of the lesion encountered at surgery. This is seemingly due to the ease of diffusion of xenon gas into the lesion.

2. Blood Flow Study

A right lateral view of a FI-Map in a healthy volunteer is illustrated in Figure 126. Usually, the high values of flow index are noted in the peripheral zone of the cerebral hemisphere and in the region of the insula or the basal ganglia.

Using 16 collimated scintillation detectors, Wilkinson and coworkers [160] also noted the high rCBF values in the periphery of the brain and in the basal ganglia region. Hilal [63] reported the densitometric study of clearance of the contrast dye in 100–150 separate regions of 2–3 mm in diameter on the rapid serial angiograms. The time course of changes in the relative quantities of the contrast dye in each region was plotted and its $T^1/_2$ value was determined. The $T^1/_2$ values were graded and the "cerebral circulation map" was drawn. The flow distribution in Hilal's study, in which the

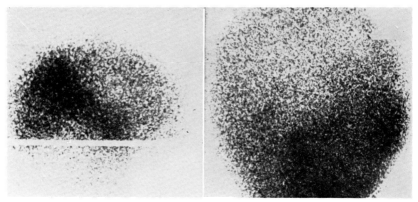

Fig. 125 Cerebral infarction. *Left:* ^{133}Xe scan, right lateral view; *Right:* ^{99m}Tc pertechnetate scan, right lateral view.

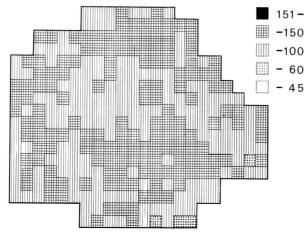

Fig. 126 Normal flow index map, left lateral view.

contrast medium is considered a flow indicator, is in essential agreement with our FI-Map.

When highly regionalized detectors are being used, it is anticipated that the distribution of the gray matter in each field differs significantly from one detector to another (Figure 127). Wilkinson and coworkers [160] evaluated the amounts of gray and white matter in each transverse rectangular block of a sliced brain. They found that the total weight of gray matter expressed as a percentage of the total weight of the cerebral hemisphere was 57 per cent gray matter, but the percentage of weight of gray matter showed a remarkable regional difference, it was high in the insular region and in the peripheral zone of the cerebral hemisphere. Thus, the regional pattern of cerebral blood flow in our study, at least in part, seems to reflect the regional difference of percentage in the weight of gray matter in each detector field. When the large differences in blood flow between the gray matter and the white matter are considered, the marked regional pattern of the flow indices is not at all surprising.

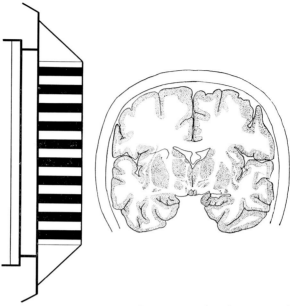

Fig. 127   Relationship of multiple detectors and the gray and white matter of the brain viewed.

Figure 128, top is a left lateral FI-Map in the patient harboring an arteriovenous malformation in the left sylvian region.   Comparing with Figure 127, it is evident that high FI values are noted in the insular region but the FI values are generally low in the other part of the brain.

Figure 129, bottom represents the washout curves in six selected ROIs in this case. There are noted in areas II, III, IV and V, the third component with very fast washout, which definitely represents the shunt peak due to arteriovenous short-circuits in the pathologic focus.

Figure 129 is the record from the patient with an arteriovenous malformation in the right parietal region.   The shaded area represents the lesion.   In areas of lesion the third component with very rapid clearance is noted, this being apparently ascribed to the arteriovenous shunt.   When the calculated $T^1/_2G$ ($T^1/_2$ of the fast component) and $T^1/_2W$ ($T^1/_2$ of the slow component) are correlated with the presence or absence of the shunt peak, it becomes evident that both $T^1/_2G$ and $T^1/_2W$ are larger in the areas where the shunt peak is noted to be present (Figure 129, right). This fact suggests that the effective cerebral blood flow is decreased in or around the arteriovenous malformation, since a large quantity of blood is by-passed through the direct arteriovenous communications in the vascular anomaly.

When 4,000 hole collimator (2.8 mm in diameter, 44.2 mm in length and 0.8 mm in thickness of septa) is used and the impulses for the NaI crystal are localized in 1,600 channel memory according to x- and y-coordination, each of 1,600 channel corresponds to the size of 5.6 mm in diameter on the crystal [61, 62].   Accordingly the count rates registered in two by two channels correspond to radioactivity for the area of 11.2 $\times$ 11.2 mm in dimension on the crystal surface.   Similarly, ROIs consisting of two by three channels correspond to 11.2 $\times$ 16.8 mm, and of three by three channels to 16.8 $\times$ 16.8 mm.

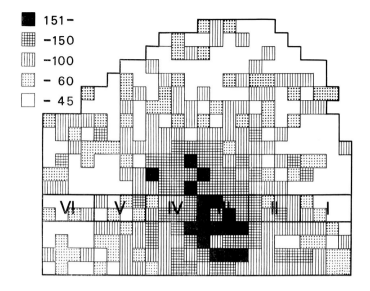

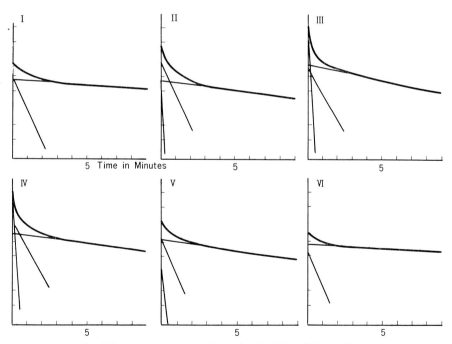

Fig. 128 Arteriovenous malformation in right sylvian region.

When two separate ^{133}Xe sources 2 mm in diameter are placed with the distance of 30 mm, two different peaks are copied on the matrix in a profile representation and between the peaks a depression by three to four channels with a markedly low count rate is obtained. When placed 20 mm apart, two active sources are copied with two peaks with a depression in between of approximately 50 per cent of the peak height.

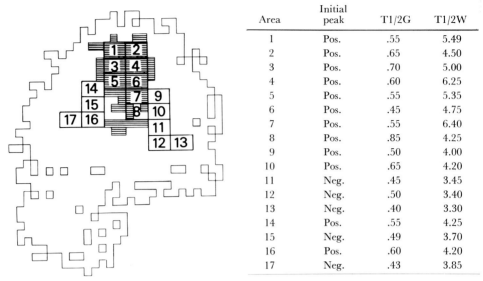

Area	Initial peak	T1/2G	T1/2W
1	Pos.	.55	5.49
2	Pos.	.65	4.50
3	Pos.	.70	5.00
4	Pos.	.60	6.25
5	Pos.	.55	5.35
6	Pos.	.45	4.75
7	Pos.	.55	6.40
8	Pos.	.85	4.25
9	Pos.	.50	4.00
10	Pos.	.65	4.20
11	Neg.	.45	3.45
12	Neg.	.50	3.40
13	Neg.	.40	3.30
14	Pos.	.55	4.25
15	Neg.	.49	3.70
16	Pos.	.60	4.20
17	Neg.	.43	3.85

Fig. 129 Arteriovenous malformation in right parietal lobe.

When the distance is decreased to 15 mm, the depression becomes less pronounced [70, 158].

Checking the collimation, the same channel on the 1,600 channel memory responded to a ^{133}Xe source of 2 mm in diameter at distances of 2, 58 and 116 mm from the scintillation camera.

From these data, we may conclude that each area of the crystal records the radioactivity from a cylinder of tissue and not from a cone, and that the dissolution is high enough for the practical use.

One drawback in the use of a scintillation camera for a rCBF measurements is the iow count rates obtained from each matrix. In an attempt to improve the accuracy, we have used the ROI with two by two, two by three, or three by three channels for calculation. From the dimensional view, the use of ROI consisting of four, six, or nine channels seems to be practical, but the count rates still remain to be of low order.

Another drawback to be pointed out here is the dead time inherent in the instrumentation. The dead time amounts to ca 2.5 μs for a Pho/Gamma III, and 12.5 μs (channel 1) to 22.5 μs (channel 39) (16.5 μs for the middle channel) for a dual ADC and a 1,600 channel memory. The transfer time from a 1,600 channel memory to a magnetic tape of 0.2 second (for 1,600 words, 10^3 characters for one word) is to be added to this. It follows that the registration obtained by this method is not the continuous but the interrupted one.

Recent availability of the data-store/playback accessory has greatly improved the technic of blood flow studies with a gamma-ray scintillation camera. The whole data of the radioactivity distribution are continuously registered on the video-tape. During the replay of the tape, the ROIs of desired size, location and form are selected. Data are directly reproduced by a dual pen-writing recorder. When ^{133}Xe is used as a tracer, the washout curve of each ROI becomes ready for immediate analysis of rCBF.

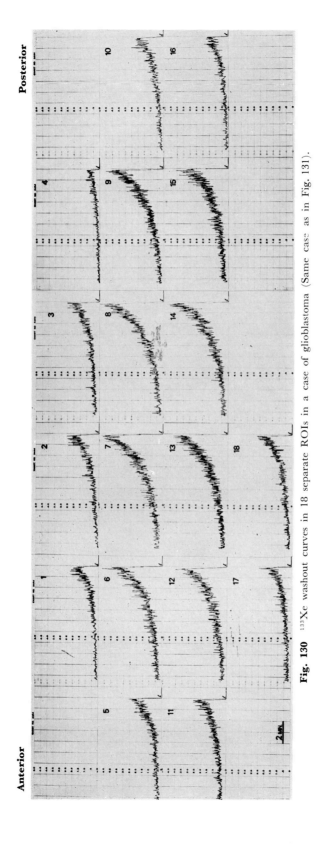

Fig. 130 ^{133}Xe washout curves in 18 separate ROIs in a case of glioblastoma (Same case as in Fig. 131).

Figure 130 is an example of the different shapes of ^{133}Xe washout curves in 18 separate portions of the brain in the patient with infiltrative glioma in the left suprasylvian region. The location and size of each of 18 ROIs as imposed on the carotid angiogram is shown in Figure 131.

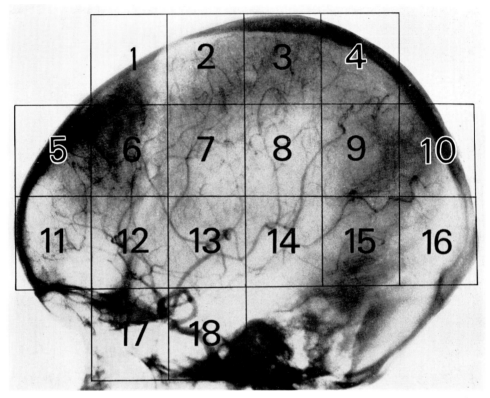

Fig. 131 Glioblastoma multiforme in left suprasylvian region. To show the sites of 18 ROIs in Fig. 130.

Figure 132 illustrates ^{133}Xe washout curves in a case of cerebral infarction. Carotid angiography showed a complete obstruction of the middle cerebral artery and stenosis of the proximal segment of the anterior cerebral artery on the right side. Five mCi of ^{133}Xe in normal saline was injected into the common carotid artery through the catheter needle used for the angiography, and washout was fed into the data-store/ playback accessory. Data of multiple separate areas of interest were replayed and recorded by pen-recorder. Markedly decreased perfusion in the territory of the involved middle cerebral artery was clearly demonstrated. Initial peak in a few areas near the base of brain seems to represent the carotid peak.

Figure 133 is the record from a case of recurrent glioblastoma multiforme in the right parieto-temporal region. Washout curves were recorded in multiple separate sites of interest. In this case, the studies were repeated under passive hyperventilation and during induced hypertension with intravenous infusion of aramine (Figure 134).

Representative curves are plotted on the semilogarithmic scale in Figure 135. The

Posterior   **Anterior**

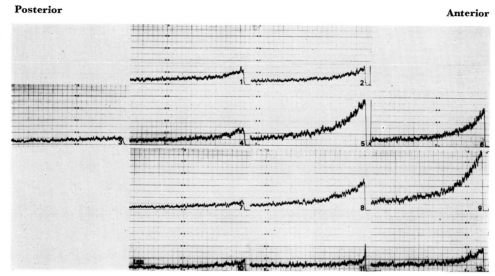

Fig. 132 ^{133}Xe washout curves in 12 ROIs in right middle cerebral occlusion.

record of area 14 (areas 6 + 10 in Figure 133) corresponds to the flow in the region of the tumor, and areas 8 and 12 represent the flow in the seemingly normal frontal brain. In the former, an increase in blood flow is evident during the hypertension, that is the autoregulation has been lost in the tumor blood flow.

Figure 136 is a record of ^{133}Xe and ^{99m}Tc pertechnetate flow studies in a case of arteriovenous malformation in the right occipital lobe. Washout curves of ^{133}Xe show the high shunt peak and a low perfusion rate in and around the site of malformation. Transit curves for various sites demonstrate the dissociation of circulatory dynamics in two different vascular beds, one in the lesion with arteriovenous shunt and the other in the normal brain.

In our experience, the data-store/playback accessory for blood flow studies has

Posterior   **Anterior**

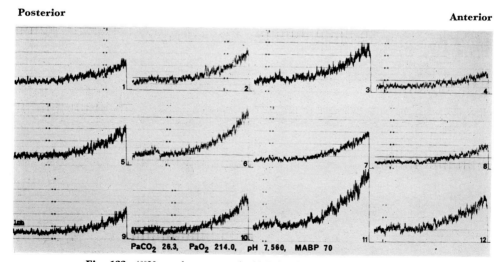

PaCO$_2$ 26.3, PaO$_2$ 214.0, pH 7.560, MABP 70

Fig. 133 ^{133}Xe washout curves in 12 ROIs in recurrent glioblastoma.

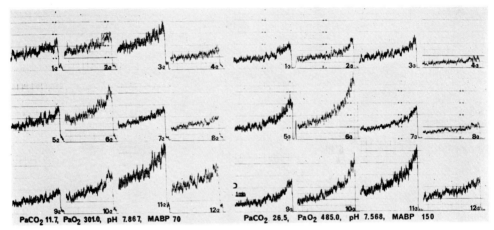

PaCO₂ 11.7, PaO₂ 301.0, pH 7.867, MABP 70   PaCO₂ 26.5, PaO₂ 485.0, pH 7.568, MABP 150

Fig. 134   [133]Xe washout curves in 12 ROIs in recurrent glioblastoma. Same case as in Fig. 133, but after hyperventilation and induced hypertension.

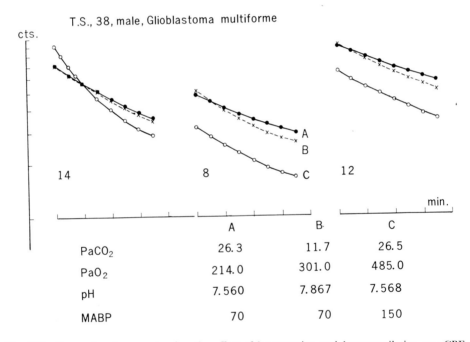

T.S., 38, male, Glioblastoma multiforme

	A	B	C
PaCO₂	26.3	11.7	26.5
PaO₂	214.0	301.0	485.0
pH	7.560	7.867	7.568
MABP	70	70	150

Fig. 135   Composite diagram showing the effect of hypertension and hyperventilation on rCBF. Same case as in Figs. 133 and 134. Area 14 represents the tumor tissue, and areas 8 and 12 seemingly normal brain.

several advantages.   Regions of interest can be selected from multiple sites of various sizes and shapes, and, after completion of the recording.   This helps greatly to avoid error in target determination, which is occasionally experienced in the blood flow studies using the multiple channel recorders.   Sequential scintigrams are obtained at the same time, which provides visual image of washout.   When the ^{133}Xe clearance study is followed by the injection of a non-diffusable tracer such as ^{99m}Tc pertechnetate, radionuclide angiograms and transit curves can be easily obtained.   Transit times can

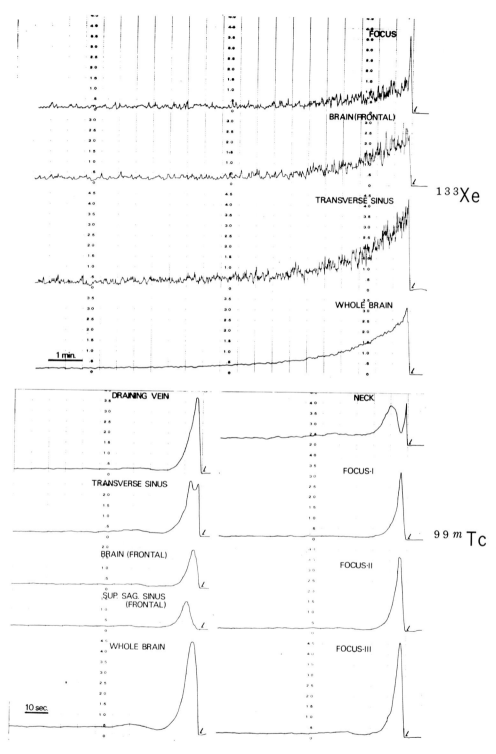

Fig. 136 ^{133}Xe washout curves and ^{99m}Tc pertechnetate tranist curves in several sites, in a case of arteriovenous malformation in the occipital lobe.

be determined for each region of interest used for ^{133}Xe studies. Furthermore, comparison with the ^{99m}Tc pertechnetate scintigram enhances the accuracy in localization of each area of interest in the ^{133}Xe studies.

Although the use of a gamma-ray scintillation camera and the data-store/playback accessory for cerebral circulation study is still in the initial stage of evolution, it is believed that the technique will be of clinical value and interest to the neurological-neurosurgical practice.

Chapter XVI

CONCLUSION

Radioisotopic brain scanning has, without question, contributed greatly to the diagnosis of organic brain disease since its introduction by Moore [105] in the late 1940s, and it has become the key screening procedure in most neurosurgical and neuroradiological centers.

The technique is quite safe and harmless, radiation to the patient is low, and the procedure is not unpleasant to the patient. Examination time of 10–20 minutes for a standard view is short so that the study can be carried out in large numbers of patients, entirely on an out-patient basis.

In recent years, newer tracers such as ^{99m}Tc pertechnetate, ^{99m}Tc DTPA, ^{113m}In DTPA or ^{169}Yb DTPA have been introduced, and together with the recent availability of the stationary image detector system, radionuclide dynamic studies (serial or sequential scintigraphy, intravenous or intra-arterial radionuclide cerebral angiography) have become possible.

Additional views such as angled posterior view, vertex view or en face view, have been introduced.

Those techniques have improved the diagnostic accuracy of brain scanning, not only on the presence or absence, and the location and size of the lesion, but also as to pathologic nature of the lesion. In addition, the use of short-lived radionuclide and the stationary image system has provided a refined experimental approach to the study of cerebral circulation in health and disease.

On the other hand, such progress in nuclear medicine may well push the brain scanning beyond the reach of the daily practice. If we use all those procedures in every patient, multiple views with multi-tracers, starting from radionuclide angiography to the delayed scan up to hours after administration and with computer display of all data, each examination takes a long time to complete and only a small number of patients can be examined within a day's work. Moreover, even with such extensive studies, brain scanning is not free of false negative cases and the procedure may still fail to be diagnostic. Limitation of the number of patients to be studied will reduce the clinical value of radioisotopic scanning as a screening procedure. In short, with a maximum effort we may lose lots and gain a minimum.

We believe, it is important to remember, in these days of rapid progress in nuclear medicine, that there are no "*routine*" scanning procedures. Each scanning schedule should be tailored to the individual case. In some patients, only the conventional scanning in the standard views may be enough for the diagnosis, in the other patients additional views may be indicated, and still in others, sequential studies including the radionuclide angiography and delayed scanning may be required for correct diagnosis.

Evidently, this approach becomes possible only with the availability of the experienced monitoring physician, who is required not only to be a nuclear radiologist but must have sufficient experience in clinical neurology and neurosurgery as well.

References

[1] ALLEN, J. N.: Extracellular space in the central nervous system. *Arch. Neurol. Psychiat.* **73:** 241, 1955.

[2] ALLEN, M. B., JR., DICK, D. A. L., HIGHTOWER, S. J., and BROWN, M.: The value and limitations of brain scanning. A review of 401 consecutive cases. *Clin. Radiol.* **18:** 19, 1966.

[3] ARONOW, S.: Positron brain scanning. *In; Progress In Medical Radioisotope Scanning*, U.S.A. E.C., Oak Ridge, 1962.

[4] BAKAY, L.: Studies in sodium exchange. Experiments with plasma, cerebrospinal fluid, and normal, injured and embryonic brain tissue. *Neurology* **10:** 564, 1960.

[5] BAKAY, L.: Basic aspects of the accumulation of substances in brain tumors. *In; Brain Tumor Scanning With Radioisotopes*, BAKAY, L., and KLEIN, D. M., Eds., Charles C. Thomas, Springfield, Ill., 1969.

[6] BALFOUR, H. H., JR., LOKEN, M. K., and BLAW, M. E.: Brain scan in a patient with herpes simplex encephalitis. *J. Pediat.* **71:** 404, 1967.

[7] BEIERWALTES, W. H., VARMA, V. M., COUNSELL, R. E., and LIEBERMAN, L. M.: Scintillation scanning of malignant melanomas with radioiodinated quinoline derivatives. *J. Nucl. Med.* **9:** 489, 1968.

[8] BINET, E. F., and LOKEN, M. K.: Scintigraphy of cerebral arteriovenous malformations and aneurysms. *Amer. J. Roentgen.* **109:** 707, 1970.

[9] BLOIS, M. S.: Melanoma detection with radioiodoquine. *J. Nucl. Med.* **9:** 492, 1968.

[10] BRINKMAN, C. A., WEGST, A. V., and KAHN, E. A.: Brain scanning with ^{203}Mercury labeled neohydrin. *J. Neurosurg.* **19:** 644, 1962.

[11] BRINKMAN, C. A., WEGST, A. B., and KAHN, E. A.: Brain scanning with mercury 203 labeled neohydrin. *J. Nucl. Med.* **6:** 687, 1965.

[12] BRIZ-KANAFANI, S., and LAZOS CONSTANTINO, G.: Perfusion ^{131}I macroaggregate brain scanning: Clinical evaluation of its diagnostic efficiency. *Amer. J. Roentgen.* **106:** 333, 1969.

[13] BRIZ-KANAFANI, S., and GARCIA-MONTEMAYOR, E.: Perfusion brain scans and the anatomic lesions encountered: A correlation. *Amer. J. Roentgen.* **109:** 686, 1970.

[14] BROWN, A. J., ZINGESSER, L., and SCHEINBERG, L. C.: Radioactive mercury labeled chlormerodrin scan in cerebral vascular accidents. *Neurology* **17:** 405, 1967.

[15] BUCY, P. C., and CIRIC, I. S.: Value of radioactive brain scans in diagnosis of brain tumors as compared with other methods. *Acta Neurochir.* **13:** 113, 1965.

[16] BUCY, P. C., and CIRIC, I. S.: Brain scans in diagnosis of brain tumors. Scanning with chlormerodrin Hg 203 and chlormerodrin Hg 197. *JAMA* **191:** 437, 1965.

[17] BUCY, P. C., and CIRIC, I. S.: Radioactive brain scans compared to other diagnostic techniques. *In; Brain Tumor Scanning With Radioisotopes*, BAKAY, L., and KLEIN, D. M., Eds., Charles C. Thomas, Springfield, Ill., 1969.

[18] BUDABIN, M.: Diagnostic value of RIHSA and chlormerodrin ^{197}Hg brain scanning in intracranial arteriovenous malformations. *J. Nucl. Med.* **8:** 879, 1967.

[19] CASTELLI, A., PAOLETTI, P., and VILLANI, R.: Brain scan for neurosurgical purposes: Analysis of 217 verified tumours. *Neurochirurgia* **11:** 234, 1968.

[20] CHEEK, W. R., and TAVERAS, J. M.: Thalamic tumors. *J. Neurosurg.* **24:** 505, 1966.

[21] CIRIC, I. S., QUINN, J. L., III., and BUCY, P. C.: Mercury 197 and technetium 99 m brain scans in the diagnosis of nonneoplastic intracranial lesions. *J. Neurosurg.* **27:** 119, 1967.

[22] COURVILLE, C. B.: *Pathology Of The Central Nervous System.* 2nd. Ed., Pacific Press, Mountain View, Calif., 1945.

[23] Cowan, R. J., Maynard, C. D., and Lassiter, K. R.: Technetium-99 m pertechnetate brain scans in the detection of subdural hematomas: A study of the age of the lesion as related to the development of a positive scan. *J. Neurosurg.* **32**: 30, 1970.

[24] Crompton, M. R.: Cerebral infarction following the rupture of cerebral berry aneurysms. *Brain* **87**: 263, 1964.

[25] Cushing, H.: *Intracranial Tumors.* Charles C. Thomas, Springfield, Ill., 1932.

[26] Cushing, H., and Eisenhardt, L.: *Meningiomas: Their Classification, Regional Behavior, Life History, And Surgical End Results.* Hafner, New York, 1962.

[27] David, R. B., Beiler, D., Hood, H., and Morrison, S. S.: Scintillation brain scanning in children. *Amer. J. Dis. Child.* **112**: 197, 1966.

[28] DeLand, F. H., and Wagner, H. N. Jr.: Brain scanning as a diagnostic aid in the detection of eighth nerve tumors. *Radiology* **92**: 571, 1969.

[29] DeLand, F. H., and Wagner, H. N. Jr.: *Atlas Of Nuclear Medicine, Vol.* **1.**, *Brain.* W. B. Saunders, Philadelphia, 1969.

[30] DiChiro, G.: RISA encephalography and conventional neuroradiologic methods. A comparative study. *Acta Radiol. (Suppl.)* **201**: 1, 1961.

[31] DiChiro, G., Ashburn, W. L., and Grove, A. S., Jr.: Which isotopes for brain scanning? *Neurology* **18**: 225, 1968.

[32] Dietz, H., Haas, J. P., and Wolf, R.: Ergebnisse der Hirntumor-diagnostik mit ^{131}I-Albumin Makroaggregaten. *Radiologe* **8**: 397, 1968.

[33] Doering, P., Krieter, G., and Lorenz, B.: Die szintigraphische Darstellung des Gehirns mit makroaggregiertem ^{131}I-Albumin. *Verh. dtsch. Ges. inn. Med.* **72**: 661, 1967.

[34] Dugger, G. S., and Pepper, F. D.: Reliability of radioisotopic encephalography: Correlation with other neuroradiological and anatomical studies. *Neurology* **13**: 1042, 1963.

[35] Economos, M., Prosalentis, A., and Leventis, A.: Value of scanning with Hg[203] in establishing histological nature of expanding intracranial processes. In; *Proc. III. Internat. Congr. Neurol. Surg.*, Excerpta Medica Foundation, Amsterdam, 1966.

[36] Filson, E. J., and Rodriguez-Antunez, A.: Isotope scanning of brain tumors using [99m]Tc. *Acta Radiol. (Diagn.)* **7**: 380, 1968.

[37] Fish, M. B., Pollycove, M., O'Reilly, S., Khentigan, A., and Kock, R. L.: Vascular characterization of brain lesions by rapid sequential cranial scintiphotography. *J. Nucl. Med.* **9**: 249, 1968.

[38] Gerhard, H., and Mundinger, F.: Biochemische Untersuchungen über Tumorspeicherung der zur Hirntumordiagnostik verwendeten Radioisotope. *Acta Radiol. (Diagn.)* **5**: 118, 1966.

[39] Gerlach, J., Jensen, H.-P., Koos, W., and Kraus, H.: *Pediatrische Neurochirurgie.* Georg Thieme, Stuttgart, 1967.

[40] Gilday, D. L., Reba, R. C., Hosain, F., Longo, R., and Wagner, H. N. Jr.: Evaluation of Ytterbium-169 diethylenetriamine-pentaacetic acid as a brain-scanning agent. *Radiology* **93**: 1129, 1969.

[41] Gilson, A. J., and Gargano, F. P.: Correlation of brain scan and angiography in intracranial trauma. *Amer. J. Roentgen.* **94**: 819, 1965.

[42] Glasgow, J. L., Currier, R. D., Goodrich, J. K., and Tutor, F. D.: Brain scans of cerebral infarcts with radioactive mercury. *Radiology* **88**: 1086, 1967.

[43]. Goodman, J. M., Mishkin, F. S., and Dyken, M.: Determination of brain death by isotope angiography. *JAMA* **209**: 1869, 1969.

[44] Goodrich, J. K., Tutor, F. T., and Webster, C. L., Jr.: The isotope encephalogram. *J. Mississippi Med. Ass.* **4**: 277, 1963.

[45]. Gotschalk, A., Aptie, J. D., Petasnick, J. P., Polcyn, R. E., and Charleston, D.B.: The comparison between sensitivity and resolution based on a clinical evaluation with the ACRIT brain scanner. *IAEA Symposium On Medical Radioisotope Scintigraphy*, Salzburg, Austria, Aug. 6–15, 1968.

[46] Gutterman, P., and Shenkin, H. A.: Cerebral scan in completed stroke. *JAMA* **207**: 145, 1969.

[47] Hagerstrand, I.: Vascular changes in cerebral metastases. *Acta Path. Microbiol. Scand.* **51**: 63, 1961.

[48] HANDA, H., HANDA, J., and EBINA, K.:   Brain scanning in cerebrovascular diseases. *Naika (Tokyo)* **22**: 1271, 1968 (*In Japanese*).

[49] HANDA, J., TAKASE, T., and HASHI, K.:   Cerebral angiography in chronic subdural hematomas; with special emphasis on the laterality of hematoma. *Brain Nerve (Tokyo)* **22**: 1271, 1968 (*In Japanese*).

[50] HANDA, J., IWAYAMA, K., YONEKAWA, Y., YOSHIDA, Y., and HANDA, H.:   The use of MAAI[131] in cerebral arteriovenous fistulas. *Amer. J. Roentgen.* **104**: 18, 1968.

[51] HANDA, J., HANDA, H., and TORIZUKA, K.:   ^{131}I-MAA in cerebral arteriovenous fistulas. *Clin. Neurol. (Tokyo)* **9**: 271, 1969 (*In Japanese*).

[52] HANDA, J., NABESHIMA, S., HANDA, H., HAMAMOTO, K., KOUSAKA, T., and TORIZUKA, K.: Serial brain scanning with technetium 99m and scintillation camera. *Amer. J. Roentgen.* **106**: 708, 1969.

[53] HANDA, J., NABESHIMA, S., HANDA, H., HAMAMOTO, K., KOUSAKA, T., and TORIZUKA, K.: Serial brain scanning by use of [99m]technetium pertechnetate and scintillation camera (PHO/GAMMA III). *Brain Nerve (Tokyo)* **21**: 1331, 1969 (*In Japanese*).

[54] HANDA, J., HANDA, H., HAMAMOTO, K., KOUSAKA, T., and TORIZUKA, K.:   Radioxenon brain scanning with gamma scintillation camera. *Brain Nerve (Tokyo)* **22**: 289, 1970 (*In Japanese*).

[55] HANDA, J., HANDA, H., TORIZUKA, K., HAMAMOTO, K., and KOUSAKA, T.:   Serial brain scanning with radioactive xenon and scintillation camera. *Amer. J. Roentgen.* **109**: 701, 1970.

[56]. HANDA, J., and HANDA, H.:   "Doughnut sign" in brain scanning. *Brain Nerve (Tokyo)* **22**: 803, 1970 (*In Japanese*).

[57] HANDA, J., HANDA, H., HAMAMOTO, K., TORIZUKA, K., and KOUSAKA, T.:   Sequential brain imaging as an aid in understanding disease etiology. *Seminars Nucl. Med.* **1**: 56, 1971.

[58] HANDA, J., HANDA, H., HAMAMOTO, K., TORIZUKA, K., and KOUSAKA, T.:   Preliminary experience on quantitative study of cerebral blood flow with gamma scintillation camera. *Brain Nerve (Tokyo)* **23**: 121, 1971 (*In Japanese*).

[59] HASEGAWA, T., RAVENS, J. R., and TOOLE, J.F.:   Precapillary arteriovenous anastomoses. "Thoroughfare channels" in brain. *Arch. Neurol. Psychiat.* **16**: 217, 1967.

[60] HEISER, W. J., QUINN, J. L., III., and MOLLIHAN, W. V.:   The crescent pattern of increased radioactivity in brain scanning. *Radiology* **87**: 483, 1966.

[61] HEISS, W.-D., PROSENZ, P., ROSZUCZKY, A., and TSCHABITSCHER, H.:   Die Verwendung von Gamma-Kamera und Vielkanalspeicher zur Messung der gesamten und regionalen Hirndurchblutung. *Nukl.-Med.* **7**: 297, 1968.

[62] HEISS, W.-D., PROSENZ, P., ROSZUCZKY, A., and TSCHABITSCHER, H.:   A quantitative gamma camera technique. *Scand. J. Lab. and Clin. Invest.*, Suppl. **102**: XI-L, 1968.

[63] HILAL, S. K.:   The regional circulation in brain tumors. *Scand. J. Lab. and Clin. Invest.*, Suppl. **102**: XV-D, 1968.

[64] HOLMES, R. A.:   The vertex view in routine brain scanning. *Amer. J. Roentgen.* **106**: 347, 1969.

[65] HOLMES, R. A., HERRON, C. S., and WAGNER, H. N., JR.:   Modified vertex view in brain scanning. *Radiology* **88**: 498, 1967.

[66] HOSAIN, F., REBA, R. C., and WAGNER, H. N., JR.:   Ytterbium-169 diethylenetriamine-pentaacetic acid complex. *Radiology* **91**: 1199, 1968.

[67] HOSSMANN, K. A.:   Morphological substrate of the blood-brain barrier in human brain tumors. *In; Brain Edema*, Klatzo, I., and SEITELBERGER, F. M., Eds., Springer, New York, 1967.

[68] HOWIESON, J., and BULL, J. W. D.:   Radiologic detection of astrocytoma involving the corpus callosum. *Amer. J. Roentgen.* **98**: 575, 1966.

[69] HUBER, P., and RÖSLER, H.:   Die Bedeutung der Angioszintigraphie in der Neuroradiologie. *Schweiz. med. Wschr.* **99**: 757, 1969.

[70] JAHNS, E.:   Vergleichende Untersuchungen der Abbildungseigenschaften bewegter und stehender Detektoren für die Szintigraphie. *In; Radioisotope In Der Lokalisationsdiagnostik.* HOFFMANN, G., and SCHEER, E., Eds., Schattauer, Stuttgart, 1967.

[71] JAMES, A. E., JR., DELAND, F. H., HODGES, F. H., III., and WAGNER, H. N., JR.: Radionuclide imaging in the detection and differential diagnosis of craniopharyngiomas. *Amer. J. Roentgen.* **109**: 692, 1970.

[72] KAHN, E. A., CROSBY, E. C., SCHNEIDER, R. C., and TAREN, J. A.: *Correlative Neurosurgery.* 2nd. Ed., Charles C. Thomas, Springfield, Ill., 1969.

[73] KENNADY, J. C., and TAPLIN, G. V.: Albumin macroaggregates for brain scanning: Experiental basis and safety in primates. *J. Nucl. Med.* **6**: 566, 1965.

[74] KERNOHAN, J. W., and UIHLEIN, A.: *Sarcomas Of The Brain.* Charles C. Thomas, Springfield, Ill., 1962.

[75] KING, E. G., WOOD, E. D., and MORLEY, T. P.: Use of macroaggregates of radioiodinated human serum albumin in brain scanning. *Canad. M. A. J.* **95**: 381, 1966.

[76] KLATZO, I., and MIQUEL, J.: Observations on pinocytosis in nervous tissue. *J. Neuropath. Exp. Neurol.* **19**: 475, 1960.

[77] KOBAYASHI, T.: The value of ^{203}Hg-neohydrin brain scan for the detection of intracranial lesions.—Relationship between positive scan and brain edema. *Brain Nerve (Tokyo)* **19**: 1221, 1967 (*In Japanese*).

[78] KRAMER, S., and ROVIT, R. L.: The value of Hg^{203} brain scans in patients with intracranial hematomas. *Radiology* **83**: 902, 1964.

[79] KRAYENBÜHL, H., and YASARGIL, M. G.: *Die Vaskulären Erkrankungen Im Gebiet Der A. Vertebralis Und A. Basilaris.* Georg Thieme, Stuttgart, 1957.

[80] LAITHA, A.: Protein metabolism of the nervous system. *Int. Rev. Neurobiol.* **6**: 1, 1964.

[81] LAWRENCE, K. M., HOARE, R. D., and TILL, K.: Diagnosis of choroid plexus papilloma of lateral ventricle. *Brain* **84**: 628, 1961.

[82] LAWRIE, B. W.: Radiology of thalamic tumors. *Clin. Radiol.* **21**: 10, 1970.

[83] LESLIE, E. V., ALKER, G. J., JR., and BAKAY, L.: The differential diagnosis of neoplastic and non-neoplastic disease on the basis of radioisotopic brain scanning. *In; Brain Tumor Scanning With Radioisotopes*, Bakay, L., and Klein, D. M., Eds., Charles C. Thomas, Springfield, Ill., 1969.

[84] LINCKE, H. D.: Radionukliduntersuchung und Szintigraphie. *In; Pädiatrische Neuroradiologie*, Decker, K., and Backmund, H., Eds., Georg Thieme, Stuttgart, 1970.

[85] LOEB, C., and MEYER, J. S.: *Strokes Due To Vertebro-basilar Disease. Infarction, Vascular Insufficiency And Hemorrhage Of The Brain Stem And Cerebellum.* Charles C. Thomas, Springfield, Ill., 1965.

[86] LOKEN, M. K., HOWELL, C., and FRENCH, L. A.: Chlormerodrin Hg 203 scintiscanning and special roentgenographic procedures. Comparison in the evaluation of brain pathology. *Arch. Neurol.* **17**: 437, 1967.

[87] LORENTZ, W. B., SEMIN, J. L., and BENNA, R. S.: Brain scanning in children. *JAMA* **201**: 5, 1967.

[88] MAHALEY, M. S., JR.: Intracranial localization of substances used for brain scanning. *Surg. Forum* **17**: 427, 1966.

[89] MANDEL, P. R., SAXE, B. I., FAEGENBURG, D., and CHIAT, H.: Demonstration of choroid plexus with technetium 99m brain scan. *Amer. J. Roentgen.* **102**: 97, 1968.

[90] MATSON, D. D.: *Neurosurgery Of Infancy And Childhood.* Charles C. Thomas, Springfield, Ill., 1969.

[91] McAFEE, G.: RISA encephalography and conventional neuroradiologic methods. *Acta Radiol. (Suppl.)* **201**: 1, 1961.

[92] McAFEE, J. G., FUEGER, C. F., STERN, H. S., WAGNER, H. N., JR., and MIGITA, T.: Tc 99m pertechnetate for brain scanning. *J. Nucl. Med.* **5**: 811, 1964.

[93] McAFEE, J. G., and FUEGER, C. F.: The values and limitation of scintillation scanning in the diagnosis of intracranial tumors. *In: Scintillation Scanning In Clinical Medicine*, Quinn, J. L., III., Ed., Saunders, Philadelphia, 1964.

[94] McAFEE, J. G., and TAXDAL, D. R.: Comparison of radioisotope scanning with cerebral angiography and air studies in brain tumor localization. *Radiology* **77**: 207, 1961.

[95] McHENRY, C. C., and VALSAMIZ, M. P.: Pathophysiology of cerebrovascular insufficiency. *G. P.* **33**: 78, 1966.

[96] McKISSOCK, W., and PAINE, K. W. E.: Primary tumors of the thalamus. *Brain* **81**: 41, 1958.

[97] MEALEY, J., JR.: Gamma-ray image of subdural effusions. Scanning after injection of radio-iodinated serum albumin into the subdural space and its clinical application. *J. Neurosurg.* **19**: 934, 1962.

[98] MEALEY, J., JR.: Brain scanning in childhood. *J. Pediat.* **69:** 399, 1966.

[99] MEALEY, J. JR., DEHNER, J. R., and REESE, I. C.: Clinical comparison of two agents used in brain scanning. Radioiodinated serum albumin vs. chlormerodrin Hg 203. *JAMA* **189:** 260, 1964.

[100] MEALEY, J., JR., and CAMPBELL, J. A.: Scintigraphy of infantile subdural effusions and its clinical application. *Acta Radiol. (Diagn.)* **5:** 871, 1966.

[101] MEALEY, J., JR., and MISHKIN, F. S.: Brain tumor scanning in children. *In: Brain Scanning With Radioisotopes,* Bakay, L., and Klein, E. M., Eds., Charles C. Thomas, Springfield, Ill., 1969.

[102] MISHKIN, F. S., and MEALEY, J., JR.: *Use And Interpretation Of The Brain Scan.* Charles C. Thomas, Springfield, Ill., 1969.

[103] MISHKIN, F. S., and DYKEN, M. L.: Increased early radionuclide activity in nasopharyngeal area in patients with internal carotid artery obstruction: "hot nose". *Radiology* **96:** 77, 1970.

[104] MOLINARI, G. F., PIRCHER, F., and HEYMAN, A.: Serial brain scanning using technetium 99m in patients with cerebral infarction. *Neurology* **17:** 627, 1967.

[105] MOORE, G. E.: Use of radioactive diiodofluorescein in the diagnosis and localization of brain tumors. *Science* **107:** 569, 1948.

[106] MORLEY, J. B., and LANGFORD, K. H.: Abnormal brain scan with subacute extradural haematomas. *J. Neurol. Neurosurg. Psychiat.* **33:** 679, 1970.

[107] MURPHY, S. E., CERVANTES, R. C., and MAASS, E. R.: Radioalbumin macroaggregate brain scanning: Histopathologic investigation. *Amer. J. Roentgen.* **102:** 88, 1968.

[108] NYSTRÖM, S.: Pathological changes in blood vessels of human glioblastoma multiforme. Comparative studies using plastic casting, angiography, light microscopy, and electron microscopy, and with reference to some other brain tumors. *Acta Path. Microbiol. Scand.* **49:** (Suppl. 137), 1960.

[109] OJEMANN, R. G., ARONOW, S., and SWEET, W. H.: Scanning with positron-emitting radioisotopes. Occlusive cerebral vascular disease. *Arch. Neurol.* **10:** 218, 1964.

[110] OJEMANN, R. G., and SWEET, W. H.: Radioisotope scanning with positron-emitting isotopes. *In; Brain Tumor Scanning With Radioisotopes.* Bakay, L., and Klein, D. M., Eds., Charles C. Thomas, Springfield, Ill., 1969.

[111] OLIVECRONA, H.: The surgical treatment of intracranial tumors. *In; Handbuch der Neurochirurgie, Vol. IV/4,* Olivecrona, H., and Tönnis, W., Eds., Springer, Berlin-Heidelberg-New York, 1967.

[112] O'MARA, R. E., MCAFEE, J. G., and CHODOC, R. B.: The "doughnut" sign in cerebral radioisotopic images. *Radiology* **92:** 581, 1969.

[113] OVERTON, M. C., III., HAYNIE, T. P., and SNODGRASS, S. R.: Brain scans in nonneoplastic intracranial lesions. Scanning with chlormerodrin Hg^{203} and chlormerodrin Hg^{197}. *JAMA* **191:** 431, 1965.

[114] OVERTON, M., C., III., OTTE, W. K., BEENTJES, L. B., and HAYNIE, T. P.: A clinical comparison of ^{197}mercury and ^{203}mercury chlormerodrin in clinical brain scanning. *J. Nucl. Med.* **6:** 28, 1965.

[115] PAUL, W., and MORLEY, T. P.: Design and function of a brain scanner for clinical use. *In; Medical Radioisotope Scanning. Vol. II.,* I.A.E.A., Vienna, 1964.

[116] PLANIOL, T.: Gamma-encephalography after ten years of utilization in neurosurgery. *In; Progress In Neurological Surgery, Vol. 1.,* KRAYENBÜHL, H., MASPES, P. E. and SWEET, W. H., Eds., S. Karger, Basel, 1966.

[117] PLANIOL, T.: Clinical experience with RISA in tumor detection. *In; Brain Tumor Scanning With Radioisotopes,* BAKAY, L., and KLEIN, D. M., Eds., Charles C. Thomas, Springfield, Ill., 1969.

[118] POTTS, D. G., and TAVERAS, J. M.: The differential diagnosis of space-occupying lesions in the region of the thalamus by cerebral angiography. *Acta Radiol. (Diagn.)* **1:** 373, 1963.

[119] QUINN, J. L., III., CIRIC, I., and HAUSER, W. N.: Analysis of 96 abnormal brain scans using Tc 99m (pertechnetate form). *JAMA* **194:** 157, 1965.

[120] RAIMONDI, A. J.: Ultrastructure and the biology of human brain tumors. *In; Progress In Neurological Surgery, Vol. 1,* KRAYENBÜHL, H., MASPES, P. E., and SWEET, W. H., Eds., S. KARGER, Basel, 1966.

[121] RAIMONDI, A. J.: Correlation of structure and function in selected tumors of the human nervous system. *Acta Neuropath.* **8:** 149, 1967.

[122] RASKIND, R., and WEISS, S. R.: Conditions simulating metastatic lesions of brain: Report of eight cases. *Internat. Surg.* **53:** 40, 1970.

[123] RASKIND, R., WEISS, S. R., MANNING, J. J., and WERMUTH, R. E.: Survival after surgical excision of single metastatic brain tumors. *Amer. J. Roentgen.* **111:** 323, 1971.

[124] RASMUSSEN, P., BUHL, J., BUSCH, H., HAASE, H., and HARMSEN, AA.: Brain scanning—Cerebral scintigraphy. An evaluation of the diagnostic value of scanning compared with other methods of investigation, based on results from 981 patients. *Acta Neurochir.* **23:** 103, 1970.

[125] RHOTON, A. L., JR.: Chlormerodrin-197Hg brain scanning. Selecting the optimal interval between isotope administration and scanning. *J. Nucl. Med.* **9:** 16, 1968.

[126] RHOTON, A. L., JR., CARLSSON, A. M., and TER-POGOSSIAN, M. M.: Posterior fossa tumors: Localization with radioactive mercury (Hg 197 or Hg 203) labeled chlormerodrin. *Arch. Neurol.* **10:** 521, 1964.

[127] RHOTON, A. L., JR., KLINKERFUSS, G. H., LILLY, D. R., and TER-POGOSSIAN, M. M.: Brain scanning in ischemic cerebrovascular disease. *Arch. Neurol.* **14:** 506, 1966.

[128] RHOTON, A. L., JR., EICHLING, J., and TER-POGOSSIAN, M. D.: Metastatic tumors: Localization by radioisotope scanning. *Neurology* **16:** 264, 1966.

[129] RÖSLER, H., and HUBER, P.: Die zerebrale Serienszintigraphie. Ergebnisse bei 208 Patienten. *Fortschritte Roentgen.* **111:** 467, 1969.

[130] RÖSLER, H., HUBER, P., and HESSE, M.: Serienszintigraphische Befunde beim Schlaganfall. *Schw. med. Wchnschr.* **100:** 1401, and 1446, 1970.

[131] ROSENTHALL, L.: Detection of altered cerebral arterial blood flow using technetium-99m pertechnetate and the gamma-ray scintillation camera. *Radiology* **88:** 713, 1967.

[132] ROSENTHALL, L.: Human brain scanning with radioiodinated macroaggregates of human serum albumin. *Radiology* **88:** 110, 1965.

[133] ROSENTHALL, L., AGUAYO, A., and STRATFORD, J.: Clinical assessment of carotid and vertebral artery injection of macroaggregates of radioiodinated albumin (MARIA) for brain scanning. *Radiology* **86:** 499, 1966.

[134] ROSENTHALL, L., MATHEWS, G., and STRATFORD, J.: Radioxenon brain scanning with the gamma-ray scintillation camera. *Radiology* **89:** 324, 1967.

[135] ROSENTHALL, L., and MARTIN, R. H.: Cerebral transit of pertechnetate given intravenously. *Radiology* **94:** 521, 1970.

[136] ROVIT, R. L., SCHECHTER, M. M., and CHORDROFF, P.: Pathology of the plexus papillomas. Observations on radiographic diagnosis. *Amer. J. Roentgen.* **110:** 608, 1970.

[137] RUSSELL, D. S., and RUBINSTEIN, L. J.: *Pathology Of The Tumors Of The Nervous System.* 2nd Ed., Williams & Wilkins, Baltimore, 1963.

[138] SCATLIFF, J. H., RADCLIFFE, W. B., PITTMAN, H. H., and PARK, C. H.: Vascular structure of glioblastomas. *Amer. J. Roentgen.* **105:** 795, 1965.

[139] SCHLESINGER, E. B., DEBOVES, S., and TAVERAS, J.: Localization of brain tumors using radioiodinated human serum albumin. *Amer. J. Roentgen.* **87:** 449, 1962.

[140] SCHMIDT, M. B.: Über die Pacchion'schen Granulationen und ihr Verhaltniss zu den Sarcomen und Psammomen der Dura Mater. *Virschow's Arch. Path. Anat.* **170:** 429, 1902.

[141] STEBNER, F. C., WILNER, H. I., and EYLER, W. R.: Correlation of pathologic and radiologic findings in brain infarction. *Radiology* **91:** 280, 1968.

[142] STÖTEBECKER, T. P.: Metastatic tumors of brain from neurosurgical point of view: Follow-up study of 158 cases. *J. Neurosurg.* **11:** 84, 1954.

[143] SWEET, W. H., and BROWNELL, G. L.: Localization of intracranial lesions by scanning with positron-emitting arsenic. *JAMA* **157:** 1183, 1955.

[144] SWEET, W. H., OJEMANN, R. G., ARONOW, S., and BROWNELL, G. L.: Radioisotopic scanning methods. I. Use of a positron emitting isotopes in the diagnosis of intracranial disease. *In; Neurologic Diagnostic Techniques,* FIELDS, W. S., Ed., Charles C. Thomas, Springfield, Ill., 1966.

[145] TAPLIN, G. V., KENNADY, J. C., GRISWOLD, M. L., and AKCAY, M. M.: Albumin 131I

macroaggregates for brain scanning. (Experimental basis and safety). *J. Nucl. Med.* **5:** 366, 1964.

[146] TATOR, C. H., MORLEY, T. P., and OLSZEWSKI, J.: A study of the factors responsible for the accumulation of radioactive iodinated serum albumin (RISA) by intracranial tumors and other-lesion. *J. Neurosurg.* **22:** 60, 1965.

[147] TATOR, C. H., and MORLEY, T. P.: Various radioactive tracers for the detection of brain tumors. *Surg. Forum* **17:** 429, 1966.

[148] TEFFT, M., JERVA, M., and MATSON, D. D.: Hg[197] chlormerodrin for brain scans in children. *Amer. J. Roentgen.* **95:** 921, 1965.

[149] TEFFT, M., MATSON, D. D., and NEUHAUSER, E. B. D.: Brain abscesses in children. Radiologic methods for early recognition. *Amer. J. Roentgen.* **98:** 675, 1966.

[150]. TOVI, D., SCHISANO, G., and LILLIEQVIST, B.: Primary tumors of the region of the thalamus. *Clin. Radiol.* **21:** 10, 1970.

[151] TRAICOFF, E., and MISHKIN, F. S.: The diagnosis of Dandy-Walker cyst by brain scanning. *Amer. J. Roentgen.* **106:** 344, 1969.

[152] UEDA, H., KITANI, K., UEDA, H., IIO, M., and KAMEDA, H.: Diagnosis of hepatic shunt by use of ^{131}I-MAA and radioiodinated gas. *Kakuigaku (Nuclear Medicine) (Tokyo)* **2:** 111, 1965 *(In Japanese)*.

[153] WAGNER, H. N., JR., HOSAIN, I., and RHODES, B. A.: Recently developed radiopharmaceuticals.: Ytterbium-169 DTPA and technetium-99m microspheres. *Radiol. Clin. North Amer.* **7:** 233, 1967.

[154] WAGNER, H. N., JR., HOSAIN, F., DELAND, F. H., and SOM, P.: A new radiopharmaceutical for cisternography: chelated Ytterbium 169. *Radiology* **95:** 121, 1970.

[155] WANG, Y.: *Clinical Radioisotope Scanning.* Charles C. Thomas, Springfield, Ill., 1967.

[156] WANG, Y., and ROSEN, J. A.: Positive brain scans in the non-space occupying lesions. *Amer. J. Roentgen.* **93:** 816, 1965.

[157] WAXMAN, H. J., SIEGLER, D. K., and RUBIN, S.: Brain scans in diagnosis of cerebrovascular disease: Scanning with Chlormerodrin Hg 203. *JAMA* **192:** 453, 1965.

[158] WESTERMAN, B. R., and GLAS, H. I.: Physical specification of a gamma camera. *J. Nucl. Med.* **9:** 24, 1968.

[159] WILCKE, O.: Results of positron scanning in 1200 cases for diagnosis of intracranial lesions. *In; Medical Radioisotope Scanning.*, Vol. II, I.A.E.A., Vienna, 1964.

[160] WILKINSON, I. M. S., BULL, J. W. D., DuBOULAY, G. H., MARSHALL, J., ROSS RUSSELL, R. W., and SYMON, L.: Regional blood flow in the normal cerebral hemisphere. *J. Neurol. Neurosurg. Psychiat.* **32:** 367, 1969.

[161] WILLIAMS, C. M., and GARCIA-BENGOCHEA, F.: Concentration of radioactive chlormerodrin in the fluid of chronic subdural haematoma. *Radiology* **84:** 745, 1965.

[162] WILLIAMS, J. L., and BEILER, D. D.: Brain scanning in nontumorous conditions. *Neurology* **16:** 1159, 1966.

[163] WILSON, E. B., and BRIGGS, R. C.: A Study of the orbital region in brain scanning, using the en face view. *Radiology* **92:** 576, 1969.

[164] WITCOFSKI, R. L., JANEWAY, R., MAYNARD, C. D., BEARDON, E. K., and SCHULTZ, J. L.: Visualization of choroid plexus in technetium 99m brain scan. *Arch. Neurol. Psychiat.* **16:** 286, 1967.

[165] WITCOFSKI, R. L., MAYNARD, C. D., and ROPER, T. J.: A comparative analysis of the accuracy of the technetium-99m pertechnetate brain scan: Followup of 1000 patients. J. *Nucl. Med.* **8:** 187, 1967.

[166] WOLPERT, S. M., HALLU, J. S., and RABE, E. F.: The value of angiography in the Dandy-Walker syndrome and posterior fossa extra-axial cysts. *Amer. J. Roentgen.* **109:** 261, 1970.

[167] WRIGHT, R. L.: Neovascularization in experimental gliomas. *J. Neuropath. Exp. Neurol.* **22:** 435, 1963.

[168] YAMAMOTO, Y. L., and FEINDEL, W. H.: Contour brain scanning and radioisotopic circulation studies for differentiating cerebrovascular lesions and tumors. *In; Brain Tumor Scanning.*, BAKAY, L., and KLEIN, D. M., Eds., Charles C. Thomas, Springfield, Ill., 1969.

[169] Zate, L. M., Hanberg, J. W., Gifford, D., and Belaz, J.: The diagnosis of tumors of the splenium of the corpus callosum. *Amer. J. Roentgen.* **101**: 130, 1967.

[170] Zingesser, L., Mandell, S., and Schechter, M.: Gamma encephalograms in extracerebral hematomas. *Acta Radiol. (Diagn.)* **5**: 972, 1966.

[171] Zülch, K. J.: *Brain Tumors: Their Biology And Pathology.* Springer, New York, 1965.

Index